INTRODUCTION

Colon cancer, also known as colorectal cancer, is a type of malignancy that originates in the colon or rectum. It is one of the most prevalent forms of cancer worldwide and a significant public health concern. Colon cancer typically begins as benign polyps on the inner lining of the colon or rectum and, over time, can transform into cancerous tumours. Various factors, including genetics, age, and lifestyle choices, influence the risk of developing colon cancer.

Diet plays a crucial role in the prevention and management of colon cancer. While no single food or dietary component can guarantee complete protection, adopting a healthful and balanced diet has been associated with a lower risk of developing this form of cancer. Several nutritional factors influence colon cancer risk, and making informed choices in one's eating habits may contribute to overall colorectal health.

1. High-Fiber Foods: Consuming a diet rich in fibre derived from whole grains, fruits, and vegetables has been linked to a reduced risk of colon cancer. Fiber aids in maintaining regular bowel movements and may help prevent the development of polyps, which can be precursors to cancer.

2. Antioxidant-Rich Foods: Fruits and vegetables, particularly those with vibrant colours, are rich in

antioxidants. These compounds help neutralize harmful free radicals in the body, potentially reducing the risk of cellular damage that could lead to cancerous growth.

3. Calcium and Vitamin D: Adequate calcium and vitamin D intake has been associated with a lower risk of colon cancer. Foods such as dairy products, leafy greens, and fatty fish can contribute to these essential nutrients, providing potential protective effects against colorectal malignancies.

4. Limitation of Red and Processed Meats: High consumption of red and processed meats has been linked to an increased risk of colon cancer. Moderating the intake of these meats and incorporating alternative protein sources may contribute to a healthier diet.

5. Healthy Fats: Choosing healthy fats, such as those found in olive oil, avocados, and nuts, can be beneficial. Limiting saturated and trans fats, often present in fried and processed foods, supports overall cardiovascular health and may have indirect benefits in colon cancer prevention.

6. Moderation in Alcohol Consumption: Excessive alcohol consumption has been associated with an elevated risk of colon cancer. Moderate and responsible alcohol consumption is recommended as part of a lifestyle that promotes colorectal health.

7. Maintaining a Healthy Weight: Being overweight or obese is a known risk factor for colon cancer. Adopting a balanced diet and engaging in regular physical activity can contribute to weight management and overall well-being.

CHAPTER ONE

What Is Colon Cancer?

Colon cancer, also known as colorectal cancer, is a malignant tumour that develops in the colon or rectum, which are parts of the large intestine. This form of cancer arises from the uncontrolled growth and division of cells in the lining of the colon or rectum, leading to the formation of polyps that can, over time, transform into cancerous tumours.

The colon, a crucial component of the digestive system, plays a vital role in absorbing water and nutrients from undigested food, while the rectum serves as a temporary storage site for faeces before elimination. Colon cancer typically originates from the inner lining of the colon or rectum, with the potential to invade nearby tissues and spread to other parts of the body, a process known as metastasis.

TYPES OF COLON CANCER

Colon cancer encompasses various types, each characterized by specific features related to the location of tumour growth, histology, and molecular characteristics. The primary types of colon cancer include:

Adenocarcinoma:

Description: Adenocarcinoma is the most common type of colon cancer, accounting for the majority of cases. It originates in the glandular cells that line the inner surface of the colon and rectum.

Characteristics: Adenocarcinomas are known for their glandular structures and can develop from precancerous polyps. These tumours may exhibit different degrees of differentiation, influencing their aggressiveness and response to treatment.

Mucinous (Colloid) Carcinoma:

Description: Mucinous carcinoma is a subtype of adenocarcinoma characterized by the presence of mucin-producing cells. These tumours have a higher proportion of mucin, a jelly-like substance, compared to other types.

Characteristics: Mucinous carcinomas are associated with a distinct appearance under the microscope and may present challenges in diagnosis and treatment due to their unique features.

Signet Ring Cell Carcinoma:

Description: Signet ring cell carcinoma is a rare and aggressive subtype of adenocarcinoma. The cells in these tumours have a characteristic appearance resembling signet rings.

Characteristics: Signet ring cell carcinomas often have a poorer prognosis compared to typical adenocarcinomas. They may be more resistant to specific treatments, emphasizing the importance of early detection and targeted interventions.

Serrated Adenocarcinoma:

Description: Serrated adenocarcinoma arises from serrated polyps, which are characterized by a saw-tooth appearance under the microscope. These polyps have been associated with an increased risk of colorectal cancer.

Characteristics: Serrated adenocarcinomas may have distinct molecular features and clinical behaviour, requiring specialized attention in diagnosis and management.

Lymphoma:

Description: Colonic lymphomas are rare cancers originating in the colon's lymphatic tissue. They can involve the colon as a primary site or be part of a systemic lymphoma.

Characteristics: Colonic lymphomas may present with symptoms such as abdominal pain, changes in bowel habits, and unexplained weight loss. Treatment involves a combination of surgery, chemotherapy, and, in some cases, radiation therapy.

CAUSES AND RISK FACTORS OF COLON CANCER

Colon cancer, like many cancers, is a complex disease influenced by a combination of genetic, environmental, and lifestyle factors. Understanding the causes and risk factors associated with colon cancer is crucial for prevention, early detection, and personalized healthcare. Here's a comprehensive overview:

Causes:

Genetic Factors:

Hereditary Syndromes: Certain inherited genetic mutations, such as those associated with Lynch syndrome and familial adenomatous polyposis (FAP), significantly increase the risk of developing colon cancer.

Age:

Increased Risk with Age: Colon cancer is more common in older individuals, with the risk rising significantly after the age of 50. However, cases can occur at any age.

Personal History:

Previous Colorectal Cancer or Polyps: Individuals with a history of colorectal cancer or certain types of polyps are at a higher risk of developing new cancers in the colon.

Inflammatory Bowel Diseases (IBD):

Ulcerative Colitis and Crohn's Disease: Chronic inflammation of the colon associated with conditions like ulcerative colitis or Crohn's disease can elevate the risk of colon cancer over time.

Family History:

First-Degree Relatives: Having a first-degree relative (parent, sibling, or child) with a history of colon cancer increases an individual's risk.

Risk Factors:

Dietary Factors:

Low-Fiber, High-Fat Diet: Diets low in fibre and high in fat, especially from red and processed meats, have been associated with an increased risk of colon cancer.

Lifestyle Choices:

Physical Inactivity: Lack of regular physical activity is linked to a higher risk of colon cancer. Regular exercise can have protective effects.

Obesity:

Increased Body Mass Index (BMI): Obesity, particularly excess abdominal fat, is a risk factor for colon cancer.

Smoking:

Tobacco Use: Smoking has been linked to an elevated risk of colon cancer, emphasizing the importance of smoking cessation for overall health.

Alcohol Consumption:

Excessive Alcohol Intake: Heavy and prolonged alcohol

consumption has been associated with an increased risk of colon cancer.

Type 2 Diabetes:

Insulin Resistance: Individuals with type 2 diabetes or insulin resistance may have an elevated risk of colon cancer.

Race and Ethnicity:

African-American Heritage: There is an increased incidence of colon cancer in African-American populations, and the reasons for this are still under investigation.

Radiation Exposure:

Previous Radiation Therapy: Individuals who have undergone radiation therapy for earlier cancers in the abdominal or pelvic area may have an increased risk.

Environmental Factors:

Exposure to Certain Chemicals: Prolonged exposure to certain industrial chemicals and pollutants may contribute to an elevated risk.

SYMPTOMS OF COLON CANCER

Colon cancer, in its early stages, often presents with subtle or no symptoms, making regular screenings crucial for early detection. As the disease progresses, symptoms may become more noticeable. Awareness of these signs is essential, as early diagnosis significantly improves the chances of successful treatment. Here are the symptoms of colon cancer:

Early Symptoms (May Be Subtle):

Changes in Bowel Habits:

Persistent diarrhoea or constipation

Changes in stool consistency or caliber

Feeling that the bowel does not empty completely

Blood in the Stool:

Visible blood in the stool

Dark, tar-like stools (melena) indicating bleeding in the upper digestive tract

Abdominal Discomfort:

Cramping or abdominal pain

Gas, bloating, or a feeling of fullness

Unexplained Weight Loss:

Unintentional weight loss without changes in diet or physical activity

Fatigue:

Persistent fatigue or weakness

Advanced Symptoms (As the Disease Progresses):

Persistent Abdominal Pain:

Ongoing or worsening abdominal pain or discomfort

Iron Deficiency Anemia:

Low red blood cell count due to chronic bleeding, leading to fatigue and weakness

Obstruction:

Bowel obstruction may cause severe abdominal pain, cramping, and an inability to pass gas or stool.

Changes in Bowel Movements:

Narrowing of the stool, often described as pencil-thin

Urgency to have a bowel movement

Weakness and Fatigue:

Generalized weakness and fatigue may accompany advanced stages of colon cancer.

Other Symptoms:

Jaundice:

Yellowing of the skin and eyes may occur if the cancer has spread to the liver.

Liver Problems:

Liver dysfunction may lead to symptoms such as abdominal swelling (ascites) or pain in the upper abdomen.

It's important to note that these symptoms can be indicative of various gastrointestinal conditions, and the presence of one or more does not necessarily confirm colon cancer. However, any persistent or unexplained symptoms should prompt a visit to a healthcare professional for further evaluation.

DIAGNOSIS OF COLON CANCER

The diagnosis of colon cancer involves a combination of medical history assessment, physical examination, and various diagnostic tests. Early detection is crucial for effective treatment and improved outcomes. Here is the diagnostic process for colon cancer:

Medical History and Physical Examination:

• Patient History: The healthcare provider will inquire about the patient's medical history, including family history of colon cancer, personal health, and any concerning symptoms.

• Physical Examination: A thorough physical examination, including a digital rectal examination (DRE), may be performed to check for signs of abnormalities.

Blood Tests:

• Complete Blood Count (CBC): A CBC can reveal abnormalities such as anaemia, which may be associated with colon cancer.

• Liver Function Tests: These tests assess the health of the liver, as colon cancer can spread to the liver.

Colonoscopy:

- Scope Examination: A colonoscopy is a primary diagnostic tool. A flexible tube with a camera (colonoscope) is inserted into the colon to examine its entire length. During the procedure, abnormal tissue samples may be collected for biopsy.

Biopsy:

- Tissue Sampling: A biopsy is performed if abnormal tissue is found during a colonoscopy. A small sample of tissue is collected and examined under a microscope to determine if cancer cells are present.

Imaging Studies:

- CT Scan: Computed tomography (CT) scans of the abdomen and pelvis may be performed to assess the extent of the cancer and check for signs of metastasis.

- MRI (Magnetic Resonance Imaging): MRI scans can provide detailed images of the colon and surrounding structures.

- PET (Positron Emission Tomography) Scan: PET scans may detect areas of increased metabolic activity, helping identify cancerous lesions.

Virtual Colonoscopy (CT Colonography):

- Non-Invasive Imaging: This procedure uses CT scans to create detailed images of the colon. While it doesn't involve a physical scope, it still requires bowel preparation.

Sigmoidoscopy:

- Partial Colon Examination: This is similar to a colonoscopy but focuses on the lower part of the colon (sigmoid colon). It may be used in certain situations but does not examine the entire colon.

Genetic Testing:

• Hereditary Risk Assessment: In cases of strong family history or when specific genetic syndromes are suspected, genetic testing may be recommended to identify specific gene mutations associated with an increased risk of colon cancer.

Staging:

• Determining the Extent: If colon cancer is diagnosed, staging is crucial. It involves specifying the extent of cancer spread, which helps guide treatment decisions. Staging may involve additional imaging studies.

Multidisciplinary Consultation:

• Team Approach: A multidisciplinary team, including oncologists, surgeons, radiologists, and pathologists, collaborates to review the diagnostic findings and develop a comprehensive treatment plan.

Second Opinion:

• Consideration: Seeking a second opinion from another healthcare professional or cancer centre is often encouraged, especially for complex cases.

COLON CANCER TREATMENT

Colon cancer treatment is a multidisciplinary approach that may involve a combination of surgery, chemotherapy, radiation therapy, immunotherapy, and targeted therapy. The specific treatment plan is tailored to the individual's diagnosis, cancer stage, overall health, and other factors.

A. Surgery:

Objective:

• Primary Tumor Removal: Surgery is often the initial treatment for colon cancer, aiming to remove the primary tumour and nearby lymph nodes.

• Stage Determination: The extent of surgical intervention depends on the cancer stage, with options ranging from local excision for early-stage tumours to colectomy (partial or complete removal of the colon) for more advanced cases.

Types of Surgical Procedures:

• Laparoscopic Surgery: Minimally invasive procedures using small incisions and a camera for visualization.

• Open Surgery: Traditional approach with a larger incision.

• Lymph Node Dissection: Removal of nearby lymph nodes to check for cancer spread.

B. Chemotherapy:

Objective:

• Systemic Treatment: Chemotherapy involves the use of drugs to destroy cancer cells throughout the body.

• Pre and Post-Surgery: Administered before surgery (neoadjuvant) to shrink tumours or after surgery (adjuvant) to eliminate remaining cancer cells.

• Control of Metastasis: Effective in treating metastatic colon cancer by targeting cancer cells that have spread to other organs.

Common Chemotherapy Drugs:

• Fluorouracil (5-FU): A cornerstone drug in colon cancer treatment.

• Oxaliplatin and Irinotecan: Often used in combination with 5-FU.

• Capecitabine: An oral alternative to 5-FU.

C. Radiation Therapy:

Objective:

• Localized Treatment: Radiation therapy uses high-energy beams to target and destroy cancer cells.

• Pre and Post-Surgery: Like chemotherapy, it can be used before surgery to shrink tumours or eliminate residual cancer cells after surgery.

• Palliative Care May be used to relieve symptoms and improve the quality of life in advanced cases.

Types of Radiation:

• External Beam Radiation: Directed at the tumour from outside the body.

• Brachytherapy: Placement of radioactive sources near or within the tumour.

D. Immunotherapy:

Objective:

• Immune System Activation: Immunotherapy aims to enhance the body's immune response against cancer cells.

• Targeting Specific Proteins: Checkpoint inhibitors like pembrolizumab and nivolumab target proteins that inhibit immune responses, allowing immune cells to attack cancer cells.

Considerations:

• Microsatellite Instability (MSI): Immunotherapy may be particularly effective in tumours with high levels of MSI.

E. Targeted Therapy:

Objective:

• Precision Treatment: Targeted therapy focuses on specific molecules involved in cancer growth, minimizing damage to normal cells.

• Blocking Growth Signals: Targeting molecules like EGFR or VEGF to hinder cancer cell growth and blood vessel formation.

Common Targeted Therapies:

• Cetuximab and Panitumumab: Target EGFR in certain cases.

• Bevacizumab and Ramucirumab: Inhibit blood vessel

formation to starve tumours of nutrients.

Multimodal Approach:

Combination Therapy:

• Customized Plans: Depending on the cancer's characteristics, treatment plans often involve a combination of the above modalities.

• Sequential Therapy: Treatment may be administered sequentially or concurrently to optimize effectiveness.

IMPORTANCE OF NUTRITION IN CANCER CARE

Nutrition plays a pivotal role in cancer care, contributing to overall health and well-being and playing a crucial role in managing treatment side effects. A well-balanced and nutrient-rich diet is essential to support the body's ability to cope with the physical and emotional challenges associated with cancer diagnosis and treatment.

1. Supporting Overall Health:

a. Immune Function:

• Adequate nutrition is vital for maintaining a robust immune system, which is critical in the body's defence against cancer cells and infections.

• Nutrient-rich foods, including fruits, vegetables, whole grains, and lean proteins, provide essential vitamins and minerals that support immune function.

b. Energy Levels:

• Cancer and its treatments can lead to fatigue and weight loss. Proper nutrition helps sustain energy levels, enabling individuals to better cope with cancer care demands.

- Balanced meals with a mix of carbohydrates, proteins, and healthy fats contribute to sustained energy throughout the day.

c. Weight Maintenance:

- Maintaining a healthy weight is essential for overall health and can positively impact treatment outcomes.

- A balanced diet helps prevent malnutrition and supports the body's ability to heal and recover.

d. Nutrient Absorption:

- Specific cancer treatments, such as surgery, radiation, or chemotherapy, can impact nutrient absorption and metabolism.

- Nutrient-dense foods help ensure that the body receives essential vitamins and minerals, even during periods of treatment-related challenges.

e. Hydration:

- Staying well-hydrated is crucial, especially during cancer treatment. Proper Hydration supports bodily functions, helps manage side effects like nausea, and aids in the elimination of toxins.

- Water-rich foods, such as fruits and vegetables, contribute to overall Hydration.

2. Managing Treatment Side Effects:

a. Nausea and Appetite Changes:

- Cancer treatments, particularly chemotherapy, can lead to nausea, changes in taste, and appetite loss.

- Eating small, frequent meals with bland and easily digestible foods can help manage these symptoms. Ginger and peppermint may also alleviate nausea.

b. Mouth and Throat Issues:

• Some cancer treatments may cause mouth sores, dry mouth, or difficulty swallowing.

• Soft, moist foods, avoiding spicy or acidic items, and staying well-hydrated can help ease discomfort and promote better nutrition.

c. Diarrhea and Constipation:

• Changes in bowel habits are common side effects of cancer treatments.

• Dietary modifications, such as increasing fibre for constipation or avoiding certain trigger foods for diarrhoea, can help regulate bowel function.

d. Muscle Wasting and Weakness:

• Cancer-related muscle wasting (cachexia) can impact physical strength and mobility.

• As tolerated, adequate protein intake and resistance exercise may help preserve muscle mass and strength.

e. Immune Support:

• Cancer treatments can suppress the immune system, increasing the risk of infections.

• Nutrient-rich foods, including those high in antioxidants and anti-inflammatory properties, can contribute to immune support and overall well-being.

CHAPTER TWO

Importance Of Nutrition In Cancer Care

Nutrition plays a pivotal role in cancer care, contributing to overall health and well-being and playing a crucial role in managing treatment side effects. A well-balanced and nutrient-rich diet is essential to support the body's ability to cope with the physical and emotional challenges associated with cancer diagnosis and treatment.

1. Supporting Overall Health:

a. Immune Function:

• Adequate nutrition is vital for maintaining a robust immune system, which is critical in the body's defence against cancer cells and infections.

• Nutrient-rich foods, including fruits, vegetables, whole grains, and lean proteins, provide essential vitamins and minerals that support immune function.

b. Energy Levels:

• Cancer and its treatments can lead to fatigue and weight loss. Proper nutrition helps sustain energy levels, enabling individuals to better cope with cancer care demands.

• Balanced meals with a mix of carbohydrates, proteins, and healthy fats contribute to sustained energy throughout the day.

c. Weight Maintenance:

• Maintaining a healthy weight is essential for overall health and can positively impact treatment outcomes.

• A balanced diet helps prevent malnutrition and supports the body's ability to heal and recover.

d. Nutrient Absorption:

• Specific cancer treatments, such as surgery, radiation, or chemotherapy, can impact nutrient absorption and metabolism.

• Nutrient-dense foods help ensure that the body receives essential vitamins and minerals, even during periods of treatment-related challenges.

e. Hydration:

• Staying well-hydrated is crucial, especially during cancer treatment. Proper Hydration supports bodily functions, helps manage side effects like Nausea, and aids in the elimination of toxins.

• Water-rich foods, such as fruits and vegetables, contribute to overall Hydration.

2. Managing Treatment Side Effects:

a. Nausea and Appetite Changes:

• Cancer treatments, particularly chemotherapy, can lead to Nausea, changes in taste, and appetite loss.

• Eating small, frequent meals with bland and easily digestible foods can help manage these symptoms. Ginger and peppermint may also alleviate Nausea.

b. Mouth and Throat Issues:

• Some cancer treatments may cause mouth sores, dry mouth, or difficulty swallowing.

• Soft, moist foods, avoiding spicy or acidic items, and staying well-hydrated can help ease discomfort and promote better nutrition.

c. Diarrhea and Constipation:

• Changes in bowel habits are common side effects of cancer treatments.

• Dietary modifications, such as increasing fibre for constipation or avoiding certain trigger foods for diarrhoea, can help regulate bowel function.

d. Muscle Wasting and Weakness:

• Cancer-related muscle wasting (cachexia) can impact physical strength and mobility.

• As tolerated, adequate protein intake and resistance exercise may help preserve muscle mass and strength.

e. Immune Support:

• Cancer treatments can suppress the immune system, increasing the risk of infections.

• Nutrient-rich foods, including those high in antioxidants and anti-inflammatory properties, can contribute to immune support and overall well-being.

DIETARY GUIDELINES FOR COLON CANCER PATIENTS

Navigating the complexities of diet is crucial for individuals diagnosed with colon cancer. Nutritional considerations play a significant role in supporting overall health and managing treatment-related side effects. Here are the dietary guidelines for colon cancer patients:

1. General Nutritional Recommendations:

a. Balanced Diet:

• Emphasize a balanced and varied diet, including a mix of fruits, vegetables, whole grains, lean proteins, and healthy fats.

• Prioritize nutrient-dense foods to meet essential vitamin and mineral needs.

b. Hydration:

• Ensure adequate Hydration, as staying well-hydrated is crucial for overall health and helps manage treatment-related side effects.

• Consume water-rich foods and beverages, and limit the Intake of caffeinated and sugary drinks.

c. Fiber Intake:

• Gradually increase dietary fibre from whole grains, fruits, and vegetables to support digestive health.

• Adapt fibre intake based on individual tolerance, especially during and after treatment, to manage potential digestive issues.

d. Lean Proteins:

• Choose lean protein sources such as poultry, fish, beans, and tofu to support muscle health and aid in recovery.

• Protein intake is vital for maintaining strength, especially during and after treatment.

e. Omega-3 Fatty Acids:

• For their anti-inflammatory properties, include sources of omega-3 fatty acids, such as fatty fish (salmon, mackerel), flaxseeds, and walnuts.

f. Portion Control:

• Practice portion control to manage weight and prevent excessive calorie intake, particularly during periods of reduced physical activity.

g. Limit Processed and Red Meats:

• Limit the consumption of processed and red meats, which may be associated with an increased risk of colon cancer.

• Choose lean cuts and consider plant-based protein alternatives.

h. Avoid Excessive Alcohol:

• Limit alcohol consumption, as excessive Intake is associated with an increased risk of colon cancer and may interfere with treatment recovery.

i. Vitamin and Mineral Supplements:

• Consult with healthcare professionals before taking supplements. In most cases, obtaining nutrients from whole foods is preferred.

• Vitamin D and calcium may be recommended for bone health, especially if there is a deficiency.

2. Adaptations during Treatment:

a. Addressing Nausea:

• Opt for bland, easily digestible foods to manage Nausea.

• Ginger, peppermint, and small, frequent meals can help ease stomach discomfort.

b. Managing Constipation and Diarrhea:

• For constipation, increase fibre gradually and stay well-hydrated.

• Avoid high-fibre and greasy foods for diarrhoea, opting for easily digestible items.

c. Maintaining Hydration:

• Consume hydrating foods like watermelon, cucumber, and soups to maintain Hydration during treatment.

• Monitor fluid intake, especially if experiencing vomiting or diarrhoea.

d. Protein Intake for Muscle Preservation:

• Prioritize protein-rich foods to preserve muscle mass during treatment-related weight changes.

• Consider protein supplements if dietary Intake needs to

be increased.

e. Soft and Moist Foods for Mouth and Throat Issues:

• For mouth sores or difficulty swallowing, choose soft, moist foods.

• Avoid hot, spicy, or acidic foods that may exacerbate discomfort.

f. Individualized Nutrition Plans:

• Work with a registered dietitian to develop a personalized nutrition plan based on individual needs, treatment phases, and specific challenges.

• Adjust the diet based on energy levels, appetite, and tolerances during different stages of treatment.

g. Immune-Boosting Foods:

• Include foods rich in antioxidants and nutrients that support the immune system, such as fruits, vegetables, and whole grains.

ROLE OF SPECIFIC NUTRIENTS IN COLON CANCER CARE

Optimal nutrition plays a crucial role in supporting individuals diagnosed with colon cancer. Specific nutrients contribute to overall health, help manage treatment-related side effects, and may even impact cancer risk. Here's a comprehensive look at the role of essential nutrients:

1. Fiber:

Role:

• Colon Health: Dietary fibre, found in fruits, vegetables, and whole grains, supports digestive health by promoting regular bowel movements and preventing constipation.

• Preventing Polyp Formation: Adequate fibre intake may reduce the risk of developing polyps, precursors to colon cancer.

Recommendations:

• Gradually increase fibre intake to prevent digestive

discomfort.

• Choose a variety of fibre-rich foods to ensure a mix of soluble and insoluble fibre.

Sources:

• Fruits: Apples, berries, pears

• Vegetables: Broccoli, carrots, spinach

• Whole Grains: Brown rice, quinoa, oats

2. Antioxidants:

Role:

• Cellular Protection: Antioxidants neutralize free radicals unstable molecules that can damage cells and contribute to cancer development.

• Immune Support: Antioxidants, such as vitamins A, C, and E, support immune function.

Recommendations:

• Consume a variety of colourful fruits and vegetables to ensure a broad spectrum of antioxidants.

• Aim for a diet rich in vitamins A, C, and E.

Sources:

• Vitamin A: Sweet potatoes, carrots, spinach

• Vitamin C: Citrus fruits, strawberries, bell peppers

• Vitamin E: Nuts, seeds, spinach

3. Omega-3 Fatty Acids:

Role:

• Anti-Inflammatory: Omega-3 fatty acids have anti-inflammatory properties, potentially reducing inflammation associated with cancer development.

• Cardiovascular Health: Supports heart health, crucial during cancer treatment.

Recommendations:

• Include fatty fish, flaxseeds, and walnuts in the diet.

• Consider omega-3 supplements under the guidance of healthcare professionals.

Sources:

• Fatty Fish: Salmon, mackerel, trout

• Plant-Based Sources: Flaxseeds, chia seeds, walnuts

4. Protein:

Role:

• Muscle Preservation: Protein is vital for maintaining muscle mass, especially during treatment-related weight changes.

• Wound Healing: Supports tissue repair and recovery after surgery or other interventions.

Recommendations:

• Include lean protein sources in every meal.

• Adjust protein intake based on individual needs and treatment phases.

Sources:

• Poultry: Chicken, turkey

• Fish: Cod, tilapia

• Plant-Based: Beans, lentils, tofu

5. Vitamins and Minerals:

Role:

• Immune Function: Vitamins and minerals, including vitamin D, vitamin C, and zinc, play crucial roles in supporting immune function.

• Bone Health: Vitamin D and calcium are essential for maintaining bone health, especially during cancer treatment.

Recommendations:

• Obtain vitamins and minerals from a well-balanced diet.

• Consider supplementation based on individual needs and deficiencies.

Sources:

• Vitamin D: Fatty fish, fortified dairy products

• Vitamin C: Citrus fruits, strawberries, bell peppers

• Calcium: Dairy products, leafy greens

• Zinc: Meat, dairy, nuts

HYDRATION IN COLON CANCER CARE

Proper Hydration is a fundamental aspect of overall health, and it holds particular significance in the context of colon cancer care. Adequate water intake plays a crucial role in supporting the body's functions, managing treatment-related side effects, and promoting well-being throughout the cancer journey.

1. Importance of Water Intake:

a. Cellular Function:

• Water is essential for various cellular functions, including nutrient transport, temperature regulation, and waste elimination.

• Hydration supports the overall health of cells, which is vital for individuals undergoing colon cancer treatment.

b. Digestive Health:

• Proper Hydration is integral to maintaining digestive health and preventing constipation, a common issue during and after cancer treatment.

• Water assists in softening stool and promoting regular bowel movements, reducing discomfort.

c. Kidney Function:

• The kidneys play a crucial role in filtering waste products from the blood. Adequate Hydration supports optimal kidney function.

• Proper water intake helps prevent kidney-related complications that may arise during specific cancer treatments.

d. Energy Levels:

• Dehydration can lead to fatigue and reduced energy levels, impacting the ability to cope with the physical and emotional challenges of cancer care.

• Staying well-hydrated supports sustained energy throughout the day.

e. Support for Treatment:

• Hydration is essential during chemotherapy, as some medications may impact kidney function or cause dehydration.

• Well-hydrated individuals may experience fewer treatment-related side effects and recover more effectively.

2. Managing Dehydration during Treatment:

a. Regular Monitoring:

• Individuals undergoing colon cancer treatment should monitor their hydration status regularly.

• Pay attention to signs of dehydration, including dark urine, dizziness, or a dry mouth.

b. Consistent Fluid Intake:

• Aim for a consistent intake of fluids throughout the day

rather than consuming large amounts at once.

• Sip water regularly, especially during meals and between treatments.

c. Adjusting for Treatment Side Effects:

• Specific cancer treatments, such as chemotherapy or radiation therapy, may increase the risk of dehydration.

• Adjust fluid Intake to account for increased needs and consult healthcare professionals for personalized recommendations.

d. Hydrating Foods:

• Incorporate water-rich foods such as watermelon, cucumbers, and soups into the diet.

• These foods contribute to overall Hydration and provide additional nutrients.

e. Electrolyte Balance:

• In cases of diarrhoea or vomiting, electrolyte imbalances can occur. Replenish electrolytes through oral rehydration solutions or foods rich in potassium and sodium.

f. Individualized Plans:

• Work with healthcare professionals, including registered dietitians, to develop individualized hydration plans.

• Factors such as age, weight, treatment type, and overall health should be considered.

g. Prevention of Nausea and Vomiting:

• Adequate Hydration can help manage Nausea and vomiting, typical side effects of cancer treatments.

• Sip on clear fluids and consume bland, easily digestible foods during periods of Nausea.

GENERAL DIETARY GUIDELINES FOR OPTIMAL HEALTH

A well-balanced and nutritious diet is a cornerstone of overall health, and it holds particular significance in promoting well-being for individuals, including those diagnosed with colon cancer. General dietary guidelines encompass a variety of food groups, each contributing essential nutrients to support overall health and aid in managing the challenges associated with colon cancer. Here are guidelines for incorporating fruits and vegetables, whole grains, lean proteins, and healthy fats into a healthy diet:

1. Fruits and Vegetables:

a. Variety is Key:

• Aim for a colourful array of fruits and vegetables to ensure a diverse range of vitamins, minerals, and antioxidants.

• Different colours often indicate other phytonutrients with unique health benefits.

b. Optimal Portions:

• Strive to fill half your plate with a variety of fruits and vegetables at each meal.

• Incorporate raw, steamed, or lightly cooked options to preserve nutrient content.

c. Fiber Intake:

• High-fibre fruits and vegetables like berries, apples, and leafy greens support digestive health.

• Gradually increase fibre intake to prevent digestive discomfort, especially during and after treatment.

d. Fresh and Seasonal Choices:

• Choose fresh, seasonal produce when possible to maximize nutrient content.

• Experiment with different cooking methods to discover flavours and textures.

2. Whole Grains:

a. Whole Grain Sources:

• Prioritize whole grains like brown rice, quinoa, oats, and whole wheat over refined grains.

• Whole grains provide fibre, vitamins, and minerals that contribute to overall health.

b. Balanced Carbohydrates:

• Incorporate whole grains into meals to provide sustained energy and support overall nutrition.

• Choose whole-grain options for bread, pasta, and cereals.

c. Portion Control:

• Be mindful of portion sizes to manage calorie intake and prevent overconsumption.

• Combine whole grains with lean proteins and vegetables for a well-balanced meal.

d. Experiment with Alternatives:

• Explore alternative whole grains like bulgur, farro, or barley to add variety to your diet.

• Experiment with recipes that incorporate diverse grains for different flavours and textures.

3. Lean Proteins:

a. Varied Protein Sources:

• Choose a variety of lean protein sources, including poultry, fish, beans, lentils, tofu, and low-fat dairy.

• Rotate protein sources to ensure a mix of essential amino acids.

b. Protein Distribution:

• Distribute protein intake evenly throughout the day to support muscle maintenance and overall health.

• Include protein-rich snacks like Greek yoghurt, nuts, or hummus.

c. Limit Processed Meats:

• Minimize the consumption of processed and red meats, which may be linked to an increased risk of colon cancer.

• Choose lean cuts and explore plant-based protein alternatives.

d. Adequate Intake:

• Ensure adequate protein intake to support immune function, wound healing, and overall recovery.

• Adjust protein levels based on individual needs, especially during and after treatment.

4. Healthy Fats:

a. Omega-3 Fatty Acids:

• Incorporate sources of omega-3 fatty acids, such as fatty fish, flaxseeds, and walnuts, for their anti-inflammatory properties.

• These fats support cardiovascular health and may contribute to overall well-being.

b. Plant-Based Fats:

• Choose healthy plant-based fats like avocados, olive oil, and nuts, which provide monounsaturated fats.

• Limit saturated and trans fats found in processed foods and certain animal products.

c. Portion Moderation:

• Practice portion control with high-fat foods to manage calorie intake.

• Opt for cooking methods that minimize added fats, such as baking, Grilling, or steaming.

d. Hydration with Healthy Fats:

• Incorporate hydrating foods rich in healthy fats, such as avocados and olive oil, to support overall Hydration.

• These fats contribute to satiety and may aid in the absorption of fat-soluble vitamins.

SAMPLE MEAL PLANS

Creating a sample meal plan for individuals, including those diagnosed with colon cancer, requires a personalized approach based on dietary preferences, nutritional needs, and any specific considerations related to the individual's health and treatment. Here's a general guide for six days of well-balanced meal plans:

Day 1:

Breakfast:

• Scrambled eggs with spinach and tomatoes

• Whole grain toast

• Fresh orange slices

Mid-Morning Snack:

• Greek yoghurt with mixed berries and a sprinkle of chia seeds

Lunch:

• Grilled chicken breast salad with mixed greens, cherry tomatoes, cucumbers, and a light vinaigrette dressing

• Quinoa on the side

Afternoon Snack:

• Sliced apples with almond butter

Dinner:

• Baked salmon with lemon and herbs

• Steamed broccoli and carrots

• Brown rice

Day 2:

Breakfast:

• Oatmeal with sliced bananas, walnuts, and a drizzle of honey

• Low-fat milk or a plant-based alternative

Mid-Morning Snack:

• A small handful of mixed nuts and a piece of string cheese

Lunch:

• Lentil soup with a side of whole-grain crackers

• Mixed vegetable salad with a light olive oil dressing

Afternoon Snack:

• Hummus with baby carrots and cherry tomatoes

Dinner:

• Grilled shrimp with a quinoa and black bean salad

• Roasted Brussels sprouts

Day 3:

Breakfast:

• Whole grain toast with avocado slices and poached eggs

• Fresh fruit salad on the side

Mid-Morning Snack:

• Cottage cheese with pineapple chunks

Lunch:

• Turkey and vegetable wrap with whole grain tortilla

• Mixed green salad with a variety of colourful veggies

Afternoon Snack:

• Greek yoghurt parfait with granola and mixed berries

Dinner:

• Baked chicken breast with rosemary and garlic

• Sweet potato wedges

• Steamed asparagus

Day 4:

Breakfast:

• Smoothie with spinach, banana, frozen berries, Greek yoghurt, and a spoon of chia seeds

• Whole grain English muffin with peanut butter

Mid-Morning Snack:

• Handful of cherry tomatoes and cucumber slices with hummus

Lunch:

• Quinoa salad with chickpeas, cherry tomatoes, red bell pepper, feta cheese, and a lemon vinaigrette

• Grilled chicken breast on the side

Afternoon Snack:

• Sliced mango with a sprinkle of Tajin seasoning

Dinner:

• Baked cod with a dill and lemon marinade

• Steamed green beans and quinoa

• Roasted sweet potato wedges

Day 5:

Breakfast:

• Avocado and tomato omelette

• Whole grain toast with butter or margarine

Mid-Morning Snack:

• Cottage cheese with sliced strawberries

Lunch:

• Whole grain pasta with tomato and vegetable sauce

• Grilled shrimp or tofu for protein

• Mixed green salad with balsamic vinaigrette

Afternoon Snack:

• Handful of almonds and a small bunch of grapes

Dinner:

• Stir-fried tofu or lean beef with broccoli, bell peppers, and snap peas

• Brown rice

Day 6:

Breakfast:

• Overnight oats with rolled oats, almond milk, chia seeds, sliced banana, and a drizzle of honey

Mid-Morning Snack:

• Apple slices with a small amount of cheese (cheddar or your preference)

Lunch:

• Spinach and arugula salad with grilled chicken, cherry tomatoes, cucumber, and a light citrus dressing

• Quinoa on the side

Afternoon Snack:

• Carrot and celery sticks with tzatziki sauce

Dinner:

• Baked tilapia with a herb and garlic crust

• Roasted Brussels sprouts and butternut squash

• Couscous

COOKING TIPS FOR COLON CANCER PATIENTS

Maintaining a healthy and well-balanced diet is essential for individuals with colon cancer. Cooking at home allows for greater control over ingredients and preparation methods. Here are crucial cooking tips with a focus on food safety and various cooking methods:

1. Food Safety:

a. Clean Hands and Surfaces:

• Wash hands thoroughly before handling food, and ensure that all utensils and surfaces are clean.

• Regularly sanitize kitchen tools and cutting boards, especially after preparing raw meats.

b. Separation of Raw and Cooked Foods:

• Prevent cross-contamination by keeping raw meats separate from ready-to-eat foods.

• Use different cutting boards for raw meats and fresh produce.

c. Temperature Control:

• Cook meats to safe internal temperatures to eliminate

harmful bacteria. Use a food thermometer to check.

• Refrigerate leftovers promptly to prevent bacterial growth.

d. Fresh Ingredients:

• Choose fresh and high-quality ingredients whenever possible.

• Be cautious with raw or undercooked eggs and seafood, especially for individuals with compromised immune systems.

e. Proper Storage:

• Store perishable foods in the refrigerator and use them within recommended time frames.

• Label leftovers with dates to track freshness.

2. Methods of Cooking:

a. Grilling:

• Grilling adds flavour without excessive added fats. Use lean cuts of meat, fish, or vegetables.

• Marinate proteins with herbs, spices, and citrus for added taste.

b. Baking and Roasting:

• Baking and roasting are healthy methods that require minimal added fats.

• Experiment with herbs and seasonings to enhance flavours.

c. Steaming:

• Steaming preserves vegetables' natural flavours and nutrients, making it a gentle cooking method.

• Steamed fish or poultry can be flavorful with added herbs and lemon.

d. Sauteing:

• Use small amounts of heart-healthy oils like olive oil for sautéing.

• Incorporate garlic, onions, and herbs for added flavour without excess salt.

e. Boiling and Simmering:

• Boil or simmer vegetables to retain their nutrients.

• Cook whole grains in simmering water for added fibre.

f. Blending and Pureeing:

• Blending or pureeing foods can provide nutritious and easily digestible options for those with difficulty chewing or swallowing.

• Create smoothies with fruits, vegetables, and protein sources for a convenient and nourishing meal.

g. Portion Control:

• Pay attention to portion sizes to avoid overeating.

• Smaller, more frequent meals can be beneficial, especially for those experiencing changes in appetite.

h. Hydration through Cooking:

• Incorporate hydrating foods like soups, stews, and broths.

• Use liquid-based cooking methods to ensure moisture retention.

i. Adapt Flavors to Preferences:

• Experiment with herbs, spices, and citrus to enhance

flavours without relying on excessive salt or sugar.

• Adjust recipes based on personal preferences to make meals enjoyable.

CHAPTER THREE

Fruits and Vegetables Recipes

Berry Blast Smoothie

Meal Description: The Berry Blast Smoothie is a vibrant and refreshing blend of antioxidant-rich berries, creating a delicious and nutrient-packed drink. This smoothie is a delightful treat for your taste buds and a nourishing addition to your day.

Ingredients:

• 1/2 cup frozen mixed berries (strawberries, blueberries, raspberries)

• 1/2 banana, frozen for a creamier texture

• 1/2 cup low-fat Greek yogurt

• 1/2 cup unsweetened almond milk

• One tablespoon of chia seeds

• One teaspoon of honey (optional for added sweetness)

• Ice cubes (optional)

Instructions:

1. Prepare Ingredients: Gather all the ingredients and ensure the berries and bananas are frozen for a cooler and thicker smoothie.

2. Blend Berries and Banana: Add the frozen mixed berries and banana in a blender.

3. Add Yogurt: Spoon in the low-fat Greek yoghurt for a creamy texture and a boost of protein.

4. Pour Almond Milk: Add the unsweetened almond milk to the blender.

5. Include Chia Seeds: Sprinkle in the chia seeds rich in omega-3 fatty acids and fibre.

6. Optional Sweetener: If desired, drizzle honey into the mix for a touch of sweetness.

7. Blend Until Smooth: Secure the blender lid and blend the ingredients until smooth and well combined.

8. Adjust Consistency: If the smoothie is too thick, add ice cubes and blend again until you achieve your desired consistency.

9. Serve Immediately: Pour the Berry Blast Smoothie into a glass and enjoy it immediately to savour its freshness.

Nutrition Information (Per Serving):

• Calories: 220

• Protein: 10g

• Fat: 6g

• Carbohydrates: 35g

• Fiber: 8g

• Sugar: 18g

MANGO AVOCADO SALAD

Meal Description: The Mango Avocado Salad is a vibrant and flavorful dish that combines the sweet and tropical essence of ripe mangoes with the creamy richness of avocados. This refreshing salad is a feast for the senses and a nutritional powerhouse, providing a mix of vitamins, healthy fats, and fibre.

Ingredients:

• Two ripe mangoes, peeled, pitted, and diced

• Two ripe avocados, peeled, pitted, and diced

• 1/2 red onion, finely chopped

• 1 cup cherry tomatoes, halved

• 1/4 cup fresh cilantro, chopped

• One jalapeño pepper, seeds removed and finely chopped (optional for heat)

• Juice of 1 lime

• Two tablespoons extra-virgin olive oil

• Salt and pepper to taste

• Mixed salad greens for serving (optional)

Instructions:

1. Prepare Ingredients: Wash, peel, pit, and dice the mangoes and avocados. Finely chop the red onion and cilantro. Halve the cherry tomatoes.

2. Combine Mango and Avocado: Gently combine the diced mangoes and avocados in a large mixing bowl.

3. Add Vegetables: Toss in the finely chopped red onion, halved cherry tomatoes, and cilantro.

4. Spice It Up (Optional): Add the finely chopped jalapeño pepper to the bowl for a hint of heat.

5. Dress with Lime Juice: Squeeze the juice of one lime over the salad to add a zesty and citrusy flavour.

6. Drizzle with Olive Oil: Pour the extra-virgin olive oil over the salad, providing a healthy dose of monounsaturated fats.

7. Season with Salt and Pepper: Season the salad with salt and pepper according to your taste preference.

8. Gently Toss: Using salad tongs or gently with your hands, toss the ingredients together until well combined, ensuring the avocado and mango are evenly coated with the lime and olive oil dressing.

9. Serve: If desired, serve the Mango Avocado Salad over a bed of mixed salad greens for added freshness.

10. Enjoy Immediately: This salad is best enjoyed immediately to relish the vibrant flavours and textures.

Nutrition Information (Per Serving):

• Calories: 250

• Protein: 3g

• Fat: 17g

- Carbohydrates: 27g
- Fiber: 9g
- Sugar: 14g

GRILLED VEGGIE SKEWERS

Meal Description: Grilled Veggie Skewers are a delightful and colourful dish that celebrates the natural flavours of assorted vegetables. This simple yet delicious recipe showcases the smoky essence of grilled veggies, making it a perfect addition to any meal or a delightful vegetarian main course.

Ingredients:

• One zucchini, sliced into rounds

• One red bell pepper, cut into chunks

• One yellow bell pepper, cut into chunks

• One red onion, quartered and separated

• 1 pint cherry tomatoes

• 8-10 button mushrooms, cleaned

• Two tablespoons of olive oil

• Two cloves garlic, minced

• One teaspoon dried oregano

• One teaspoon of dried thyme

• Salt and pepper to taste

• Wooden skewers, soaked in water for 30 minutes

Instructions:

1. Prepare Vegetables: Wash and chop zucchini, red and yellow bell peppers, red onion, cherry tomatoes, and mushrooms into bite-sized pieces.

2. Marinate Vegetables: In a bowl, combine olive oil, minced garlic, dried oregano, dried thyme, salt, and pepper. Add the prepared vegetables to the marinade, ensuring they are well-coated. Let them marinate for at least 15-20 minutes.

3. Assemble Skewers: Thread the marinated vegetables onto the soaked wooden skewers, alternating between different veggies for a colourful presentation.

4. Preheat Grill: Preheat the grill to medium-high heat.

5. Grill Skewers: Place the assembled veggie skewers on the preheated grill. Grill for 10-15 minutes, turning occasionally, until the vegetables are tender and have a nice char.

6. Baste with Marinade (Optional): Baste the skewers with any remaining marinade during the grilling process for added flavour.

7. Check for Doneness: Ensure that the vegetables are cooked to your preferred level of doneness. They should be tender but still have a slight crispness.

8. Serve: Remove the grilled veggie skewers from the grill and transfer them to a serving platter. Serve immediately.

Nutrition Information (Per Serving):

• Calories: 120

• Protein: 3g

• Fat: 7g

- Carbohydrates: 14g
- Fiber: 4g
- Sugar: 7g

SPINACH AND STRAWBERRY SALAD

Meal Description: The Spinach and Strawberry Salad is a delightful blend of fresh, crisp spinach leaves paired with the sweetness of ripe strawberries. This refreshing salad not only tantalizes the taste buds but also provides a burst of vitamins, minerals, and antioxidants, making it a perfect addition to any meal.

Ingredients:

• 6 cups fresh baby spinach leaves, washed and dried

• 1 cup strawberries, hulled and sliced

• 1/2 cup feta cheese, crumbled

• 1/4 cup red onion, thinly sliced

• 1/4 cup chopped pecans or walnuts (optional for crunch)

• Balsamic vinaigrette dressing (homemade or store-bought)

• Salt and pepper to taste

Instructions:

1. Prepare Ingredients: Wash and thoroughly dry the

baby spinach leaves. Hull the strawberries and slice them into halves or quarters. Crumble the feta cheese and thinly slice the red onion.

2. Assemble Salad Base: In a large salad bowl, combine the fresh spinach leaves, sliced strawberries, crumbled feta cheese, and thinly sliced red onion.

3. Add Nuts (Optional): For added crunch and texture, sprinkle chopped pecans or walnuts over the salad.

4. Season with Salt and Pepper: Lightly season the salad with salt and pepper to taste. Be mindful of the salt content in the dressing.

5. Drizzle with Dressing: Just before serving, drizzle the desired amount of balsamic vinaigrette dressing over the salad. Toss gently to coat the ingredients evenly.

6. Serve Immediately: Transfer the Spinach and Strawberry Salad to individual serving plates or bowls. Serve immediately to enjoy the freshness of the ingredients.

Nutrition Information (Per Serving):

• Calories: 180

• Protein: 7g

• Fat: 12g

• Carbohydrates: 15g

• Fiber: 4g

• Sugar: 7g

CITRUS INFUSED QUINOA SALAD

Meal Description: The Citrus Infused Quinoa Salad is a vibrant and zesty dish that combines the wholesome goodness of quinoa with the refreshing flavours of citrus fruits. Packed with colourful vegetables, this salad is a nutritional powerhouse, offering a delightful mix of textures and tastes.

Ingredients:

• 1 cup quinoa, rinsed and cooked according to package instructions

• One orange, segmented

• One grapefruit, segmented

• One cucumber, diced

• One red bell pepper, diced

• 1/4 cup red onion, finely chopped

• 1/4 cup fresh cilantro or mint, chopped

• 1/4 cup feta cheese, crumbled (optional)

• Two tablespoons extra-virgin olive oil

• Juice of 1 lemon

• Salt and pepper to taste

Instructions:

1. Cook Quinoa: Rinse the quinoa under cold water and cook it according to package instructions. Once cooked, let it cool to room temperature.

2. Prepare Citrus Segments: Peel the orange and grapefruit, removing the white pith. Segment the citrus fruits by carefully cutting out the individual sections.

3. Dice Vegetables: Dice the cucumber and red bell pepper into small, bite-sized pieces. Finely chop the red onion.

4. Assemble Salad Base: In a large bowl, combine the cooked quinoa, citrus segments, diced cucumber, diced red bell pepper, and chopped red onion.

5. Add Fresh Herbs: Sprinkle fresh cilantro or mint over the salad for a burst of herbaceous flavour.

6. Optional Feta Cheese: Add crumbled feta cheese for a creamy and tangy element if desired.

7. Prepare Citrus Dressing: In a small bowl, whisk together extra-virgin olive oil, lemon juice, salt, and pepper to create a citrus-infused dressing.

8. Drizzle Dressing: Pour the citrus dressing over the salad and toss gently to ensure all ingredients are evenly coated.

9. Chill (Optional): For enhanced flavours, refrigerate the salad for at least 30 minutes before serving.

10. Serve: Transfer the Citrus Infused Quinoa Salad to a serving platter or individual bowls. Garnish with additional herbs or feta if desired. Serve and enjoy!

Nutrition Information (Per Serving):

• Calories: 250

- Protein: 8g
- Fat: 10g
- Carbohydrates: 35g
- Fiber: 6g
- Sugar: 6g

ROASTED VEGETABLE MEDLEY

Meal Description: The Roasted Vegetable Medley is a delightful and nutritious dish that brings out the natural flavours of a variety of vegetables through the caramelization process of roasting. This colourful and savoury medley is visually appealing and a versatile side dish that complements a range of main courses.

Ingredients:

- 2 cups baby potatoes, halved

- Two carrots, peeled and sliced into rounds

- One zucchini, sliced

- One red bell pepper, cut into chunks

- One yellow bell pepper, cut into chunks

- One red onion, cut into wedges

- Two tablespoons of olive oil

- Two cloves garlic, minced

- One teaspoon of dried thyme

- One teaspoon of dried rosemary

• Salt and pepper to taste

• Fresh parsley for garnish (optional)

Instructions:

1. Preheat Oven: Preheat your oven to 425°F (220°C).

2. Prepare Vegetables: Wash, peel, and chop the baby potatoes, carrots, zucchini, red and yellow bell peppers, and red onion.

3. Toss with Olive Oil and Seasonings: In a large bowl, toss the prepared vegetables with olive oil, minced garlic, dried thyme, dried rosemary, salt, and pepper. Ensure all vegetables are well coated.

4. Arrange on Baking Sheet: Spread the seasoned vegetables in a single layer on a baking sheet. Ensure there's space between the pieces for even roasting.

5. Roast in the Oven: Place the baking sheet in the preheated oven and roast for 25-30 minutes or until the vegetables are tender and have a golden brown colour, stirring halfway through.

6. Check for Doneness: Test the vegetables with a fork to ensure they are cooked to your desired level of tenderness.

7. Garnish (Optional): Garnish the Roasted Vegetable Medley with fresh parsley for a burst of colour and additional flavour.

8. Serve: Transfer the roasted vegetables to a serving platter. Serve as a side dish alongside your favourite main course, or enjoy them on their own.

Nutrition Information (Per Serving):

• Calories: 180

- Protein: 3g
- Fat: 8g
- Carbohydrates: 25g
- Fiber: 5g
- Sugar: 6g

PINEAPPLE CUCUMBER SALSA

Meal Description: The Pineapple Cucumber Salsa is a refreshing and tropical twist on a classic salsa. This vibrant medley of flavours combines the sweetness of ripe pineapple with the crispness of cucumber, creating a versatile salsa that pairs perfectly with grilled proteins, tacos, or as a delightful dip for tortilla chips.

Ingredients:

• 1 cup fresh pineapple, finely diced

• One cucumber peeled, seeded, and finely diced

• 1/4 cup red onion, finely chopped

• One jalapeño pepper, seeds removed and finely diced

• 1/4 cup fresh cilantro, chopped

• Juice of 1 lime

• Salt and pepper to taste

• Optional: 1 avocado, diced, for added creaminess

Instructions:

1. Prepare Ingredients: Dice the fresh pineapple, cucumber, red onion, jalapeño pepper, and cilantro. If using avocado, dice it into small pieces.

2. Combine Ingredients: In a mixing bowl, combine the

diced pineapple, cucumber, red onion, jalapeño pepper, and cilantro. If using avocado, gently fold it in to avoid mashing.

3. Squeeze Lime Juice: Squeeze the juice of one lime over the mixture. Adjust the amount to your taste preference.

4. Season with Salt and Pepper: Sprinkle salt and pepper over the salsa, adjusting the seasoning according to your taste.

5. Mix Well: Gently toss the ingredients together until well combined, ensuring an even distribution of flavours.

6. Chill (Optional): For enhanced flavours, refrigerate the salsa for at least 30 minutes before serving.

7. Serve: Transfer the Pineapple Cucumber Salsa to a serving bowl. Serve it as a topping for grilled chicken or fish, a side dish, or a refreshing dip for tortilla chips.

Nutrition Information (Per Serving):

• Calories: 40

• Protein: 1g

• Fat: 0g

• Carbohydrates: 10g

• Fiber: 2g

• Sugar: 6g

MIXED BERRY PARFAIT

Meal Description: The Mixed Berry Parfait is a delightful and visually appealing dessert that layers the goodness of fresh berries with creamy yoghurt and a hint of sweetness. This parfait is a treat for the taste buds and a nutritious and antioxidant-rich way to satisfy your sweet cravings.

Ingredients:

• 1 cup mixed berries (strawberries, blueberries, raspberries)

• 1 cup Greek yoghurt (vanilla or plain)

• Two tablespoons of honey or maple syrup

• 1/2 cup granola

• Fresh mint leaves for garnish (optional)

Instructions:

1. Prepare Berries: Wash and hull strawberries. If using larger berries, cut them into bite-sized pieces.

2. Sweeten Yogurt: Mix Greek yoghurt with honey or maple syrup in a bowl, adjusting sweetness to your preference.

3. Assemble Parfait:

• Begin by placing a layer of mixed berries at the bottom of serving glasses or bowls.

• Add a layer of sweetened Greek yoghurt on top of the berries.

• Sprinkle a layer of granola over the yoghurt.

• Repeat the layers until the glasses are filled, finishing with a layer of berries on top.

1. Garnish (Optional): Garnish the top with a few fresh mint leaves for a burst of colour and added freshness.

2. Serve Immediately: Serve the Mixed Berry Parfait immediately to enjoy the contrast of textures and temperatures.

3. Variations:

• Nutty Crunch: Add a layer of chopped nuts (such as almonds or walnuts) between the yoghurt and granola for extra crunch.

• Layer with Seeds: Sprinkle chia seeds or flaxseeds between the layers for added nutritional benefits.

1. Customize to Taste: Feel free to adjust the quantities of berries, yoghurt, and granola based on personal preferences.

Nutrition Information (Per Serving):

• Calories: 250

• Protein: 12g

• Fat: 8g

• Carbohydrates: 35g

• Fiber: 5g

• Sugar: 18g

STUFFED BELL PEPPERS WITH QUINOA AND BLACK BEANS

Meal Description: These Stuffed Bell Peppers with Quinoa and Black Beans are a nutritious and flavorful dish that combines the goodness of quinoa, black beans, and vibrant bell peppers. Packed with protein, fibre, and a medley of vegetables, this meal is satisfying and a visually appealing centrepiece for a wholesome dinner.

Ingredients:

• Four large bell peppers (any colour), halved and seeds removed

• 1 cup quinoa, rinsed and cooked

• One can (15 oz) black beans, drained and rinsed

• 1 cup corn kernels (fresh, frozen, or canned)

• 1 cup diced tomatoes

• 1/2 cup red onion, finely chopped

• Two cloves garlic, minced

• One teaspoon of ground cumin

- One teaspoon of chilli powder
- Salt and pepper to taste
- 1 cup shredded Mexican blend cheese (optional)
- Fresh cilantro or green onions for garnish
- Lime wedges for serving

Instructions:

1. Preheat Oven: Preheat your oven to 375°F (190°C).
2. Prepare Bell Peppers: Cut the bell peppers in half lengthwise, removing the seeds and membranes. Lightly brush the outsides with olive oil if desired.
3. Cook Quinoa: Rinse the quinoa under cold water and cook it according to package instructions.
4. Prepare Filling:
5. Combine cooked quinoa, black beans, corn, diced tomatoes, red onion, minced garlic, ground cumin, chilli powder, salt, and pepper in a large bowl. Mix well.
6. Stuff Bell Peppers:
7. Stuff each bell pepper half with the quinoa and black bean mixture, pressing down gently to pack the filling.
8. Optional Cheese Topping:
9. If desired, sprinkle shredded Mexican blend cheese over the stuffed peppers.
10. Bake in the Oven:
11. Place the stuffed bell peppers in a baking dish. Bake for 25-30 minutes or until the peppers are tender.

12. Broil for a Crispy Top (Optional):
13. If you prefer a crispy cheese top, broil for an additional 2-3 minutes until the cheese is golden and bubbly.
14. Garnish and Serve:
15. Remove from the oven and garnish with fresh cilantro or green onions. Serve with lime wedges on the side.
16. Enjoy! Serve these Stuffed Bell Peppers hot, and enjoy a nutritious, plant-based meal.

Nutrition Information (Per Serving):

• Calories: 300

• Protein: 14g

• Fat: 5g

• Carbohydrates: 55g

• Fiber: 10g

• Sugar: 6g

CAULIFLOWER AND BROCCOLI STIR-FRY

Meal Description: This Cauliflower and Broccoli Stir-Fry is a quick, flavorful, and nutritious dish that highlights the natural goodness of two cruciferous vegetables. The stir-fry is enhanced with a savoury soy-based sauce, making it a delicious and satisfying option for a wholesome meal.

Ingredients:

• One small head of cauliflower, cut into florets

• One medium-sized broccoli crown cut into florets

• One carrot, julienned

• One bell pepper (any colour), thinly sliced

• Three cloves garlic, minced

• One tablespoon of fresh ginger, grated

• Two tablespoons of soy sauce

• One tablespoon of oyster sauce (optional for umami flavour)

• One tablespoon of sesame oil

• One tablespoon vegetable oil (for cooking)

• One tablespoon cornstarch (optional for a thicker sauce)

• Sesame seeds and chopped green onions for garnish

• Cooked brown rice or quinoa for serving

Instructions:

Prepare Vegetables:

Wash and cut cauliflower and broccoli into bite-sized florets.

Julienne the carrot and thinly slice the bell pepper.

Prepare Sauce:

Mix soy sauce, oyster sauce (if using), sesame oil, and cornstarch (if desiring a thicker sauce). Set aside.

Stir-Fry:

Heat vegetable oil in a large pan or wok over medium-high heat.

Add minced garlic and grated ginger. Stir-fry for about 30 seconds until fragrant.

Add Vegetables:

Add cauliflower, broccoli, julienned carrot, and sliced bell pepper to the pan. Stir-fry for 4-5 minutes until the vegetables are slightly tender but still crisp.

Sauce It Up:

Pour the prepared sauce over the vegetables. Toss and stir to coat the vegetables evenly. Cook for an additional 2-3 minutes.

Check for Doneness:

Taste a piece of cauliflower or broccoli to check for desired doneness. The vegetables should be tender yet have a slight crunch.

Serve:

Remove the pan from heat. Serve the Cauliflower and Broccoli Stir-Fry over cooked brown rice or quinoa.

Garnish:

Garnish with sesame seeds and chopped green onions for added flavour and visual appeal.

Enjoy!

Serve this delicious stir-fry immediately and enjoy a wholesome and flavorful meal.

Nutrition Information (Per Serving, without rice/quinoa):

• Calories: 150

• Protein: 6g

• Fat: 9g

• Carbohydrates: 15g

• Fiber: 5g

• Sugar: 5g

CHAPTER FOUR

Whole Grains Recipes

Brown Rice Pilaf With Almonds

Brown Rice Pilaf with Almonds

Meal Description: Brown Rice Pilaf with Almonds is a wholesome and flavorful dish that combines the nutty goodness of brown rice with the crunch of toasted almonds. This simple yet delicious recipe transforms basic brown rice into a delectable side dish that pairs well with a variety of main courses.

Ingredients:

• 1 cup brown rice

• 2 cups vegetable or chicken broth

• 1/4 cup slivered almonds

• One small onion, finely chopped

• Two cloves garlic, minced

• Two tablespoons of olive oil

• One teaspoon of dried thyme

• One teaspoon of dried parsley

• Salt and pepper to taste

• Fresh parsley for garnish (optional)

Instructions:

Rinse Brown Rice: Rinse the brown rice under cold water until the water runs clear.

Toast Almonds:

Over medium heat, toast the slivered almonds in

a dry skillet until they are golden brown and fragrant. Stir frequently to prevent burning. Once toasted, set aside.

Sauté Onion and Garlic:

In a saucepan, heat olive oil over medium heat. Add finely chopped onion and minced garlic. Sauté until the onion is translucent and aromatic.

Add Brown Rice:

Stir in the brown rice, coating it with the onion and garlic mixture. Cook for 1-2 minutes to lightly toast the rice.

Add Broth and Herbs:

Pour the vegetable or chicken broth, and add dried thyme and parsley. Season with salt and pepper to taste. Bring the mixture to a boil.

Simmer and Cook:

Reduce the heat to low, cover the saucepan with a lid, and simmer for 40-45 minutes or until the rice is tender and has absorbed the liquid. Stir occasionally.

Fluff and Add Almonds:

Once the rice is cooked, fluff it with a fork. Stir in the toasted slivered almonds, ensuring an even distribution.

Garnish and Serve:

Garnish the Brown Rice Pilaf with fresh parsley if desired. Serve as a flavorful side dish alongside your favourite proteins.

Enjoy!

Enjoy this nutty and wholesome Brown Rice Pilaf with Almonds as part of a well-balanced meal.

Nutrition Information (Per Serving):

• Calories: 220

• Protein: 5g

• Fat: 9g

• Carbohydrates: 32g

• Fiber: 4g

• Sugar: 1g

QUINOA AND CHICKPEA STUFFED TOMATOES

Meal Description: Quinoa and Chickpea Stuffed Tomatoes are a flavorful, protein-packed dish that transforms fresh tomatoes into a delicious, wholesome meal. This recipe combines Quinoa's nutty texture, chickpeas's creaminess, and a medley of herbs and spices to create a satisfying and nutritious stuffing.

Ingredients:

• Four large tomatoes

• 1 cup cooked Quinoa

• One can (15 oz) chickpeas, drained and rinsed

• 1/2 cup red onion, finely chopped

• 1/2 cup cucumber, diced

• 1/4 cup fresh parsley, chopped

• Two tablespoons of olive oil

• One tablespoon of lemon juice

• One teaspoon of ground cumin

• One teaspoon paprika

• Salt and pepper to taste

• Feta cheese crumbles for garnish (optional)

Instructions:

Preheat Oven: Preheat your oven to 375°F (190°C).

Prepare Tomatoes:

Cut the tops off the tomatoes and scoop out the seeds and pulp, creating a hollow cavity. You can use a spoon to remove the inner part of the tomatoes carefully.

Prepare Quinoa and Chickpea Mixture:

Combine cooked Quinoa, chickpeas, finely chopped red onion, diced cucumber, fresh parsley, olive oil, lemon juice, ground cumin, paprika, salt, and pepper in a bowl. Mix well.

Stuff Tomatoes:

Generously stuff each tomato with the quinoa and chickpea mixture, pressing down gently to pack the stuffing.

Bake:

Place the stuffed tomatoes in a baking dish. Bake in the preheated oven for 20-25 minutes or until the tomatoes are tender.

Optional Cheese Topping:

If desired, sprinkle feta cheese crumbles over the stuffed tomatoes during the last 5 minutes of baking for a creamy finish.

Check for Doneness:

Ensure the tomatoes are cooked to your desired

level of tenderness.

Serve:

Remove from the oven and let them cool for a few minutes. Serve the Quinoa and chickpea-stuffed tomatoes as a light and nutritious main course or side dish.

Garnish (Optional):

Garnish with additional fresh parsley and feta cheese crumbles if desired.

Enjoy!

Enjoy this wholesome and flavorful dish as part of a balanced meal.

Nutrition Information (Per Serving):

• Calories: 250

• Protein: 10g

• Fat: 8g

• Carbohydrates: 35g

• Fiber: 8g

• Sugar: 5g

OATMEAL WITH BERRIES AND NUTS

Meal Description: Oatmeal with Berries and Nuts is a wholesome and nourishing breakfast that combines the heartiness of oats with the sweetness of berries and the crunch of nuts. This comforting dish provides a balanced mix of fibre, vitamins, and healthy fats to kickstart your day on a nutritious note.

Ingredients:

• 1 cup old-fashioned oats

• 2 cups milk (dairy or plant-based)

• 1 cup mixed berries (strawberries, blueberries, raspberries)

• 1/4 cup chopped nuts (almonds, walnuts, or your choice)

• One tablespoon of honey or maple syrup

• 1/2 teaspoon vanilla extract

• Pinch of salt

• Greek yoghurt for topping (optional)

Instructions:

Cook Oats:

Bring the milk to a gentle simmer in a saucepan

over medium heat.

Stir in the old-fashioned oats and a pinch of salt.

Reduce heat to low and simmer, stirring occasionally, until the oats are cooked to your desired consistency (usually about 5-7 minutes).

Add Sweetener and Vanilla:

Stir in honey or maple syrup and vanilla extract. Adjust the sweetness to your liking.

Prepare Berries:

Wash and prepare the mixed berries. If using larger berries like strawberries, slice them into bite-sized pieces.

Toast Nuts:

In a separate dry skillet over medium heat, toast the chopped nuts until they are golden and fragrant. Stir frequently to prevent burning.

Assemble Oatmeal:

Spoon the cooked oats into bowls.

Top with a generous portion of mixed berries and toasted nuts.

Optional Yogurt Topping:

Add a dollop of Greek yoghurt on top for added creaminess and protein.

Drizzle with Honey (Optional):

If desired, drizzle a little extra honey or maple syrup over the oatmeal for sweetness.

Serve and Enjoy!

Serve the Oatmeal with Berries and Nuts warm, and enjoy a comforting and nutritious breakfast.

Nutrition Information (Per Serving):

- Calories: 350

- Protein: 12g

- Fat: 12g

- Carbohydrates: 50g

- Fiber: 8g

- Sugar: 15g

WHOLE WHEAT PASTA PRIMAVERA

Meal Description: Whole Wheat Pasta Primavera is a vibrant and nutrient-packed dish that celebrates the freshness of seasonal vegetables with the wholesome goodness of whole wheat pasta. This colourful and flavorful pasta dish is delicious and provides a healthy dose of fibre, vitamins, and minerals.

Ingredients:

- 8 oz whole wheat pasta

- Two tablespoons of olive oil

- Three cloves garlic, minced

- One onion, thinly sliced

- One carrot, julienned

- One bell pepper (any colour), thinly sliced

- One zucchini, thinly sliced

- 1 cup cherry tomatoes, halved

- 1 cup broccoli florets, blanched

- 1/2 cup snap peas, trimmed

- 1/4 cup fresh basil, chopped

- 1/4 cup grated Parmesan cheese

- Salt and pepper to taste
- Red pepper flakes for a spicy kick (optional)

Instructions:

Cook Whole Wheat Pasta:

Cook the whole wheat pasta according to the package instructions until al dente. Drain and set aside.

Sauté Garlic and Onions:

In a large skillet, heat olive oil over medium heat. Add minced garlic and thinly sliced onions. Sauté until the onions are translucent and the garlic is fragrant.

Add Vegetables:

Add julienned carrots, thinly sliced bell pepper, zucchini, cherry tomatoes, blanched broccoli florets, and snap peas to the skillet. Stir-fry for 5-7 minutes or until the vegetables are tender-crisp.

Season and Toss:

Season the vegetables with salt and pepper to taste. If you enjoy a bit of heat, add red pepper flakes. Toss the vegetables to combine.

Combine with Pasta:

Add the cooked whole wheat pasta to the skillet with the sautéed vegetables. Toss everything together until well combined.

Finish with Fresh Basil and Parmesan:

Stir in chopped fresh basil and grated Parmesan cheese. Toss to incorporate the flavours.

Serve:

Transfer the Whole Wheat Pasta Primavera to serving plates. Optionally, garnish with additional Parmesan and fresh basil.

Enjoy!

Serve immediately and savour this delicious and nutritious Whole Wheat Pasta Primavera.

Nutrition Information (Per Serving):

• Calories: 400

• Protein: 15g

• Fat: 10g

• Carbohydrates: 65g

• Fiber: 12g

• Sugar: 8g

BARLEY AND VEGETABLE SOUP

Meal Description: Barley and Vegetable Soup is a hearty and nutritious dish that combines barley's wholesome goodness with an array of colourful vegetables. Packed with fibre, vitamins, and minerals, this comforting soup is not only delicious but also a satisfying way to enjoy a variety of nutrient-dense ingredients.

Ingredients:

- 1 cup pearl barley, rinsed

- One tablespoon of olive oil

- One onion, diced

- Two carrots diced

- Two celery stalks, diced

- Two cloves garlic, minced

- One zucchini, diced

- 1 cup green beans, chopped

- One can (15 oz) diced tomatoes

- 8 cups vegetable broth

- One teaspoon of dried thyme

- One teaspoon of dried rosemary

• Salt and pepper to taste

• Fresh parsley for garnish

Instructions:

Prepare Barley:

Rinse the pearl barley under cold water. Set aside.

Sauté Aromatics:

In a large pot, heat olive oil over medium heat. Add diced onion, carrots, and celery. Sauté until the vegetables are softened.

Add Garlic and Vegetables:

Add minced garlic to the pot and sauté for an additional minute. Then, add diced zucchini and chopped green beans to the pot.

Incorporate Tomatoes and Barley:

Pour in the diced tomatoes with their juices. Add the rinsed pearl barley to the pot. Stir to combine.

Pour in Vegetable Broth:

Pour in the vegetable broth, ensuring that the barley is fully submerged. Bring the soup to a gentle boil.

Season and Simmer:

Season the soup with dried thyme, dried rosemary, salt, and pepper. Reduce the heat to low, cover the pot, and simmer for about 45-60 minutes or until the barley is tender.

Adjust Seasoning:

Taste the soup and adjust the seasoning if necessary. Add more salt and pepper to suit your preference.

Garnish and Serve:

Ladle the Barley and Vegetable Soup into bowls. Garnish with fresh parsley for a burst of colour and freshness.

Enjoy!

Serve this nourishing Barley and Vegetable Soup hot, and enjoy a comforting and wholesome meal.

Nutrition Information (Per Serving):

• Calories: 250

• Protein: 8g

• Fat: 4g

• Carbohydrates: 50g

• Fiber: 12g

• Sugar: 8g

FARRO AND ROASTED VEGETABLE BOWL

Meal Description: The Farro and Roasted Vegetable Bowl is a wholesome and satisfying dish that combines Farro's chewy texture with the rich flavours of roasted vegetables. This nutrient-packed bowl offers a variety of colours, textures, and flavours, making it a delightful and nutritious choice for a balanced meal.

Ingredients:

• 1 cup farro, rinsed

• 2 cups vegetable broth

• One sweet potato, peeled and cubed

• One red bell pepper, sliced

• One zucchini, sliced

• One red onion, thinly sliced

• Two tablespoons of olive oil

• One teaspoon of dried thyme

• One teaspoon of smoked paprika

• Salt and pepper to taste

- 1 cup cherry tomatoes, halved

- 1/4 cup feta cheese, crumbled (optional)

- Fresh parsley for garnish

Instructions:

Prepare Farro:

In a saucepan, combine rinsed Farro and vegetable broth. Bring to a boil, then reduce heat, cover, and simmer for about 25-30 minutes or until the Farro is tender but still has a chewy texture. Drain any excess liquid.

Preheat Oven:

Preheat the oven to 400°F (200°C).

Roast Vegetables:

On a baking sheet, toss sweet potato cubes, sliced red bell pepper, zucchini slices, and thinly sliced red onion with olive oil, dried thyme, smoked paprika, salt, and pepper. Spread the vegetables in a single layer.

Roast in the Oven:

Roast the vegetables in the preheated oven for 25-30 minutes or until they are tender and slightly caramelized, stirring halfway through. Add cherry tomatoes in the last 5 minutes of roasting.

Assemble the Bowl:

In serving bowls, layer the cooked Farro and top it with the roasted vegetables, including the cherry tomatoes.

Optional Feta Cheese:

If desired, sprinkle crumbled feta cheese over the bowl for added creaminess.

Garnish and Serve:

Garnish the Farro and Roasted Vegetable Bowl with fresh parsley for a burst of colour and freshness.

Enjoy!

Serve this wholesome bowl immediately, savouring the combination of nutty Farro and flavorful roasted vegetables.

Nutrition Information (Per Serving):

• Calories: 400

• Protein: 10g

• Fat: 10g

• Carbohydrates: 70g

• Fiber: 12g

• Sugar: 8g

BULGUR SALAD WITH POMEGRANATE SEEDS

Meal Description: Bulgur Salad with Pomegranate Seeds is a refreshing and vibrant dish that combines the nutty flavour of Bulgur with the sweet and tart pop of pomegranate seeds. This salad is a delicious and nutritious addition to your menu, packed with fibre, antioxidants, and a medley of fresh herbs.

Ingredients:

- 1 cup coarse Bulgur
- 2 cups boiling water
- 1 cup pomegranate seeds
- One cucumber, diced
- One red bell pepper, diced
- 1/2 red onion, finely chopped
- 1/4 cup fresh mint leaves, chopped
- 1/4 cup fresh parsley, chopped
- 1/4 cup extra-virgin olive oil

- Two tablespoons of lemon juice
- One teaspoon of ground cumin
- Salt and pepper to taste
- Feta cheese crumbles for garnish (optional)

Instructions:

Prepare Bulgur:

Place coarse Bulgur in a bowl and pour boiling water over it. Cover the bowl and let it sit for about 20-30 minutes or until the Bulgur has absorbed the water and becomes tender. Fluff with a fork.

Combine Ingredients:

In a large mixing bowl, combine the soaked Bulgur, pomegranate seeds, diced cucumber, diced red bell pepper, finely chopped red onion, chopped fresh mint leaves, and chopped fresh parsley.

Prepare Dressing:

Whisk together extra-virgin olive oil, lemon juice, ground cumin, salt, and pepper in a small bowl to create the dressing.

Toss and Dress:

Pour the dressing over the bulgur mixture and toss everything together until well coated.

Chill (Optional):

For enhanced flavours, refrigerate the Bulgur Salad for at least 30 minutes before serving.

Garnish and Serve:

Garnish the salad with feta cheese crumbles if desired.

Enjoy!

Serve this delightful Bulgur Salad with Pomegranate Seeds as a light, satisfying side dish or standalone meal.

Nutrition Information (Per Serving):

• Calories: 300

• Protein: 7g

• Fat: 15g

• Carbohydrates: 40g

• Fiber: 10g

• Sugar: 8g

MULTI-GRAIN PANCAKES WITH BLUEBERRIES

Meal Description: Multi-Grain Pancakes with Blueberries are a wholesome and delicious breakfast option that combines the goodness of various grains with the burst of flavour from fresh blueberries. These hearty pancakes are a treat for your taste buds and provide a nutritious start to your day.

Ingredients:

- 1/2 cup whole wheat flour

- 1/4 cup oats

- 1/4 cup cornmeal

- Two tablespoons of buckwheat flour

- One tablespoon of ground flaxseed

- One teaspoon of baking powder

- 1/2 teaspoon baking soda

- 1/4 teaspoon salt

- 1 cup buttermilk (or milk of choice)

- One large egg

• Two tablespoons melted butter or oil

• One tablespoon of maple syrup or honey

• One teaspoon of vanilla extract

• 1/2 cup fresh blueberries

• Cooking spray or additional butter for cooking

Instructions:

Prepare Dry Ingredients:

Whisk together whole wheat flour, oats, cornmeal, buckwheat flour, ground flaxseed, baking powder, baking soda, and salt in a large bowl.

Prepare Wet Ingredients:

Whisk together buttermilk, egg, melted butter or oil, maple syrup or honey, and vanilla extract in a separate bowl.

Combine Wet and Dry Ingredients:

Pour the wet ingredients into the dry ingredients and stir until just combined. Do not overmix; a few lumps are okay.

Add Blueberries:

Gently fold in fresh blueberries into the pancake batter.

Preheat Griddle or Pan:

Preheat a griddle or non-stick pan over medium heat. Lightly coat with cooking spray or butter.

Cook Pancakes:

Pour 1/4 cup of batter for each pancake onto the griddle. Cook until bubbles form on the surface, then flip and cook the other side until golden brown.

Keep Warm:

Keep the cooked pancakes warm in a low oven while you make the remaining ones.

Serve:

Serve the Multi-Grain Pancakes with Blueberries with additional blueberries, maple syrup, or your favourite toppings.

Enjoy!

Enjoy these wholesome and flavorful pancakes for a nutritious breakfast.

Nutrition Information (Per Serving, two pancakes):

• Calories: 300

• Protein: 8g

• Fat: 12g

• Carbohydrates: 40g

• Fiber: 6g

• Sugar: 8g

WHOLE GRAIN WRAPS WITH TURKEY AND AVOCADO

Meal Description: Whole Grain Wraps with Turkey and Avocado are nutritious and satisfying for a quick and wholesome meal. Packed with lean protein, healthy fats, and fibre, these wraps offer a balanced combination of flavours and textures that make for a delicious and guilt-free lunch or dinner.

Ingredients:

• Four whole-grain wraps

• 1 pound sliced turkey breast

• One large avocado, sliced

• 1 cup cherry tomatoes, halved

• 1 cup mixed greens (spinach, arugula, or your choice)

• 1/2 red onion, thinly sliced

• 1/4 cup Greek yoghurt or your favourite dressing

• One tablespoon of Dijon mustard

• Salt and pepper to taste

Instructions:

Prepare Ingredients:

Wash and prepare all the fresh ingredients. Slice the turkey breast, avocado, cherry tomatoes, and red onion.

Warm Wraps (Optional):

If desired, warm the whole grain wraps in a dry skillet for a few seconds on each side or according to package instructions.

Assemble Wraps:

Lay out the whole-grain wraps on a clean surface.

Spread a thin layer of Dijon mustard on each wrap.

Layer Ingredients:

Place a generous portion of sliced turkey breast on each wrap.

Add avocado slices, halved cherry tomatoes, mixed greens, and thinly sliced red onion.

Drizzle Dressing:

Drizzle Greek yoghurt or your favourite dressing over the ingredients. Season with salt and pepper to taste.

Fold and Roll:

Fold the sides of each wrap and then roll them up tightly, creating a secure wrap.

Slice and Serve:

If desired, slice the wraps in half at a diagonal angle for easier handling.

Serve immediately.

Enjoy!

Enjoy these Whole Grain Wraps with Turkey and Avocado as a wholesome and flavorful meal.

Nutrition Information (Per Serving, one wrap):

• Calories: 350

• Protein: 25g

• Fat: 15g

• Carbohydrates: 30g

• Fiber: 8g

• Sugar: 4g

WILD RICE AND MUSHROOM RISOTTO

Meal Description: Wild Rice and Mushroom Risotto is a hearty and flavorful dish that combines the nutty goodness of wild rice with the earthy richness of mushrooms. This variation of classic risotto is not only delicious but also a nutritious choice for a comforting and satisfying meal.

Ingredients:

• 1 cup wild rice

• 3 cups vegetable or chicken broth

• Two tablespoons of olive oil

• One onion, finely chopped

• Two cloves garlic, minced

• 8 oz mixed mushrooms (such as cremini, shiitake, or oyster), sliced

• 1 cup Arborio rice

• 1/2 cup dry white wine

• One teaspoon of fresh thyme leaves

• 1/2 cup grated Parmesan cheese

• Salt and black pepper to taste

• Fresh parsley for garnish

Instructions:

Cook Wild Rice:

In a separate pot, cook the wild rice according to package instructions. This typically involves rinsing the rice, combining it with water, and simmering until tender. Drain any excess water.

Prepare Broth:

Heat the vegetable or chicken broth in a saucepan and keep it warm over low heat.

Sauté Onion and Garlic:

Heat olive oil over medium heat in a large skillet or wide saucepan. Add finely chopped onion and sauté until translucent. Add minced garlic and cook for an additional minute.

Cook Mushrooms:

Add sliced mushrooms to the skillet and cook until they release their moisture and become golden brown.

Add Arborio Rice:

Stir in Arborio rice and cook for 2-3 minutes, allowing the rice to toast slightly.

Deglaze with White Wine:

Pour in the dry white wine to deglaze the pan. Stir until the rice mainly absorbs the wine.

Add Thyme and Broth:

Sprinkle fresh thyme leaves over the rice. Begin

adding the warm broth, one ladle at a time, stirring frequently. Wait until the liquid is mostly absorbed before adding the next ladle of broth.

Continue Cooking:

Continue this process until the Arborio rice is cooked to al dente, creamy, and has a slight bite. This typically takes about 18-20 minutes.

Fold in Wild Rice and Parmesan:

Once the Arborio rice is cooked, fold in the cooked wild rice and grated Parmesan cheese. Stir until well combined.

Season and Garnish:

Season the risotto with salt and black pepper to taste. Garnish with fresh parsley.

Serve:

Serve the Wild Rice and Mushroom Risotto immediately, and enjoy this comforting and flavorful dish.

Nutrition Information (Per Serving):

• Calories: 350

• Protein: 10g

• Fat: 8g

• Carbohydrates: 60g

• Fiber: 5g

• Sugar: 2g

CHAPTER FIVE

Lean Proteins Recipes

Grilled Salmon With Dill Sauce

Meal Description: Grilled Salmon with Dill Sauce is a delicious and healthy dish that combines the rich flavour of grilled salmon with the freshness of a tangy dill sauce. This recipe is a feast for the senses and provides a generous dose of omega-3 fatty acids and essential nutrients.

Ingredients:

• Four salmon fillets (6 oz each), skin-on

• Two tablespoons of olive oil

• One teaspoon of lemon zest

• Two tablespoons of lemon juice

• Two cloves garlic, minced

• Salt and black pepper to taste

• Fresh dill for garnish

Dill Sauce:

• 1/2 cup Greek yogurt

• Two tablespoons mayonnaise

• One tablespoon of fresh dill, finely chopped

• One tablespoon of capers, drained and chopped

• One teaspoon of Dijon mustard

• Salt and black pepper to taste

Instructions:

Preheat Grill:

Preheat the grill to medium-high heat.

Prepare Salmon:

Pat the salmon fillets dry with paper towels. Mix olive oil, lemon zest, lemon juice, minced garlic, salt, and black pepper in a small bowl to create a marinade.

Marinate Salmon:

Brush the salmon fillets with the marinade, ensuring they are evenly coated. Let them marinate for 15-20 minutes to allow the flavours to infuse.

Grill Salmon:

Place the salmon fillets on the preheated grill, skin-side down. Grill for about 4-5 minutes per side or until the salmon is cooked through and has grill marks. The internal temperature should reach 145°F (63°C).

Prepare Dill Sauce:

Whisk together Greek yoghurt, mayonnaise, finely chopped dill, capers, Dijon mustard, salt, and black pepper in a small bowl. Adjust the seasoning to your taste.

Serve:

Transfer the grilled salmon fillets to serving plates. Drizzle each fillet with a generous spoonful of the dill sauce.

Garnish:

Garnish the Grilled Salmon with Dill Sauce with

additional fresh dill.

Enjoy!

Serve immediately and savour the succulent grilled salmon with the zesty dill sauce.

Nutrition Information (Per Serving):

• Calories: 350

• Protein: 30g

• Fat: 22g

• Carbohydrates: 5g

• Fiber: 1g

• Sugar: 2g

BAKED CHICKEN BREAST WITH LEMON AND HERBS

Meal Description: Baked Chicken Breast with Lemon and Herbs is a simple yet flavorful dish that showcases the natural taste of chicken enhanced by the brightness of lemon and the aromatic blend of herbs. This easy-to-make recipe results in tender and juicy chicken breasts with a burst of citrusy and herby goodness.

Ingredients:

• Four boneless, skinless chicken breasts

• Two tablespoons of olive oil

• Zest of 1 lemon

• Juice of 1 lemon

• Two cloves garlic, minced

• One teaspoon of dried thyme

• One teaspoon of dried rosemary

• One teaspoon dried oregano

• Salt and black pepper to taste

• Fresh parsley for garnish

Instructions:

Preheat Oven:

Preheat the oven to 400°F (200°C).

Prepare Chicken:

Pat the chicken breasts dry with paper towels. Place them in a baking dish.

Create Marinade:

Whisk together olive oil, lemon zest, lemon juice, minced garlic, dried thyme, rosemary, dried oregano, salt, and black pepper in a small bowl.

Marinate Chicken:

Pour the marinade over the chicken breasts, ensuring they are evenly coated. Allow the chicken to marinate for at least 15-20 minutes to absorb the flavours.

Bake:

Bake the chicken breasts in the preheated oven for 20-25 minutes or until the internal temperature reaches 165°F (74°C). The cooking time may vary based on the thickness of the chicken breasts.

Check for Doneness:

To check for doneness, insert a meat thermometer into the thickest part of the chicken. It should register 165°F (74°C), and the juices should run clear.

Garnish:

Sprinkle freshly chopped parsley over the baked chicken for a burst of colour and freshness.

Rest and Serve:

Allow the chicken to rest for a few minutes before serving. This helps retain its juices and ensures a tender texture.

Serve:

Serve the Baked Chicken Breast with Lemon and Herbs with your favourite side dishes or a light salad.

Enjoy!

Enjoy this simple and delightful dish featuring the natural flavours of chicken, enhanced by the bright and herby combination of lemon and herbs.

Nutrition Information (Per Serving):

• Calories: 250

• Protein: 30g

• Fat: 12g

• Carbohydrates: 2g

• Fiber: 1g

• Sugar: 0g

TURKEY AND VEGETABLE STIR-FRY

Meal Description: Turkey and Vegetable Stir-Fry is a quick and nutritious dish that combines lean ground turkey with a colourful assortment of vegetables, all stir-fried to perfection. This recipe offers a balance of protein, fibre, and vitamins, making it a delicious and wholesome option for a speedy weeknight dinner.

Ingredients:

- 1 pound ground turkey
- Two tablespoons of soy sauce
- One tablespoon of oyster sauce
- One tablespoon of sesame oil
- Two tablespoons of vegetable oil
- Three cloves garlic, minced
- One tablespoon of fresh ginger, grated
- One red bell pepper, thinly sliced
- One yellow bell pepper, thinly sliced
- 1 medium carrot, julienned

- 1 cup snap peas, trimmed
- 1 cup broccoli florets
- Two green onions, sliced (for garnish)
- Sesame seeds (optional, for garnish)
- Cooked brown rice or quinoa (for serving)

Instructions:

Prepare Sauce:

Mix soy sauce, oyster sauce, and sesame oil in a small bowl to create the stir-fry sauce.

Cook Ground Turkey:

In a large wok or skillet, heat vegetable oil over medium-high heat. Add minced garlic and grated ginger, sautéing for about 30 seconds until fragrant.

Add ground turkey to the wok, breaking it apart with a spatula. Cook until the turkey is browned and cooked through.

Add Vegetables:

Add sliced red and yellow bell peppers, julienned carrot, snap peas, and broccoli florets to the wok. Stir-fry for 3-4 minutes until the vegetables are tender-crisp.

Pour in Sauce:

Pour the prepared stir-fry sauce over the turkey and vegetables. Stir to coat evenly and let it simmer for an additional 1-2 minutes.

Check Seasoning:

Taste and adjust the seasoning if needed. You can

add a bit more soy sauce or sesame oil, according to your preference.

Garnish and Serve:

Garnish the Turkey and Vegetable Stir-Fry with sliced green onions and, if desired, sprinkle with sesame seeds.

Serve Over Rice or Quinoa:

Serve the stir-fry over cooked brown rice or quinoa.

Enjoy!

Enjoy this delicious and wholesome Turkey and Vegetable Stir-Fry as a satisfying and flavorful meal.

Nutrition Information (Per Serving, without rice/quinoa):

- Calories: 300

- Protein: 25g

- Fat: 15g

- Carbohydrates: 15g

- Fiber: 5g

- Sugar: 5g

VEGETARIAN LENTIL SOUP

Meal Description: Vegetarian Lentil Soup is a hearty and nutritious dish that combines the earthy flavour of lentils with an assortment of vegetables and aromatic spices. This comforting soup is delicious and packed with protein, fibre, and essential nutrients.

Ingredients:

- 1 cup dried green or brown lentils, rinsed and drained
- One tablespoon of olive oil
- One onion, diced
- Two carrots diced
- Two celery stalks, diced
- Three cloves garlic, minced
- One can (14 oz) diced tomatoes
- 6 cups vegetable broth
- One teaspoon of ground cumin
- One teaspoon of ground coriander
- One teaspoon of smoked paprika
- 1/2 teaspoon turmeric
- One bay leaf

• Salt and black pepper to taste

• 2 cups spinach or kale, chopped

• Juice of 1 lemon

• Fresh parsley for garnish

Instructions:

Prepare Lentils:

Rinse and drain the lentils. Set aside.

Sauté Aromatics:

In a large pot, heat olive oil over medium heat. Add diced onion, carrots, and celery. Sauté until the vegetables are softened.

Add Garlic and Spices:

Add minced garlic to the pot and sauté for an additional minute. Stir in ground cumin, ground coriander, smoked paprika, turmeric, and a bay leaf.

Incorporate Lentils and Tomatoes:

Add the rinsed lentils to the pot, followed by diced tomatoes. Stir to combine with the aromatic vegetables and spices.

Pour in Vegetable Broth:

Pour in the vegetable broth, ensuring that the lentils are fully submerged. Bring the soup to a gentle boil.

Season and Simmer:

Season the soup with salt and black pepper to taste. Reduce the heat to low, cover the pot, and let it simmer for about 25-30 minutes or until the lentils are tender.

Add Leafy Greens:

Stir in chopped spinach or kale and let it wilt into the soup.

Finish with Lemon Juice:

Squeeze the juice of one lemon into the soup. Stir to combine.

Adjust Seasoning:

Taste the soup and adjust the seasoning if necessary. Add more salt, pepper, or lemon juice to suit your preference.

Garnish and Serve:

Garnish the Vegetarian Lentil Soup with fresh parsley.

Enjoy!

Serve this wholesome and flavorful soup hot, and enjoy a nourishing bowl of Vegetarian Lentil Soup.

Nutrition Information (Per Serving):

• Calories: 250

• Protein: 15g

• Fat: 5g

• Carbohydrates: 40g

• Fiber: 15g

• Sugar: 5g

CHICKPEA AND SPINACH CURRY

Meal Description: Chickpea and Spinach Curry is a delicious and wholesome plant-based dish that combines protein-rich chickpeas with vibrant spinach in a flavorful curry sauce. This quick and easy recipe is packed with nutrients and bursting with aromatic spices that make it a comforting and satisfying meal.

Ingredients:

- Two cans (15 oz each) of chickpeas, drained and rinsed

- One tablespoon of vegetable oil

- One onion, finely chopped

- Three cloves garlic, minced

- One tablespoon of fresh ginger, grated

- One can (14 oz) diced tomatoes

- One can (14 oz) coconut milk

- Two teaspoons of curry powder

- One teaspoon of ground cumin

- One teaspoon of ground coriander

- 1/2 teaspoon turmeric

- 1/2 teaspoon cayenne pepper (adjust to taste)

- Salt and black pepper to taste
- 6 cups fresh spinach, chopped
- Juice of 1 lime
- Fresh cilantro for garnish
- Cooked basmati rice (for serving)

Instructions:

Sauté Aromatics:

In a large skillet or pot, heat vegetable oil over medium heat. Add chopped onion and sauté until softened.

Add Garlic and Ginger:

Add minced garlic and grated ginger to the skillet. Sauté for an additional minute until fragrant.

Incorporate Spices:

Stir in curry powder, ground cumin, ground coriander, turmeric, and cayenne pepper. Cook the spices for 1-2 minutes to enhance their flavours.

Add Chickpeas:

Add drained and rinsed chickpeas to the skillet. Stir to coat them with the aromatic spice mixture.

Pour in Tomatoes and Coconut Milk:

Pour in diced tomatoes (with their juices) and coconut milk. Season with salt and black pepper to taste. Stir well to combine.

Simmer:

Allow the curry to simmer over medium-low heat for about 15-20 minutes, allowing the flavours to meld and the chickpeas to absorb the curry sauce.

Add Spinach:

Just before serving, stir in chopped fresh spinach and let it wilt into the curry.

Finish with Lime Juice:

Squeeze the juice of one lime into the curry. Stir to combine.

Adjust Seasoning:

Taste the curry and adjust the seasoning if necessary. Add more salt, pepper, or lime juice to suit your preference.

Garnish and Serve:

Garnish the Chickpea and Spinach Curry with fresh cilantro.

Serve Over Rice:

Serve the curry over cooked basmati rice.

Enjoy!

Enjoy this flavorful and nutritious Chickpea and Spinach Curry as a delightful plant-based meal.

Nutrition Information (Per Serving, without rice):

- Calories: 300

- Protein: 10g

- Fat: 15g

- Carbohydrates: 35g

- Fiber: 12g

- Sugar: 5g

TOFU AND VEGETABLE SKEWERS

Meal Description: Tofu and Vegetable Skewers are a delightful and nutritious way to enjoy the goodness of plant-based ingredients. These skewers feature marinated tofu cubes paired with colourful vegetables, creating a visually appealing and flavorful dish. Whether you grill them or bake them in the oven, these skewers are a tasty addition to your vegetarian repertoire.

Ingredients:

• One block of extra-firm tofu pressed and cut into cubes

• One zucchini, sliced into rounds

• One bell pepper (any colour), cut into chunks

• One red onion, cut into chunks

• Cherry tomatoes

• Wooden skewers soaked in water for at least 30 minutes

Marinade:

• Three tablespoons soy sauce

• Two tablespoons of olive oil

• Two tablespoons maple syrup or agave nectar

- Two cloves garlic, minced
- One teaspoon of ground cumin
- One teaspoon of smoked paprika
- Salt and black pepper to taste

Instructions:

Prepare Marinade:

Whisk together soy sauce, olive oil, maple syrup or agave nectar, minced garlic, ground cumin, smoked paprika, salt, and black pepper in a bowl.

Marinate Tofu:

Gently toss the tofu cubes in half of the marinade, ensuring they are well coated. Allow the tofu to marinate for at least 30 minutes to absorb the flavours.

Preheat Grill or Oven:

Preheat your grill or oven to medium-high heat.

Assemble Skewers:

Thread the marinated tofu cubes, zucchini slices, bell pepper chunks, red onion chunks, and cherry tomatoes onto the soaked wooden skewers in an alternating pattern.

Brush with Marinade:

Brush the skewers with the remaining marinade for an extra burst of flavour.

Grill or Bake:

Grill the skewers for 10-15 minutes, turning occasionally, until the tofu is golden brown and the vegetables are tender. Alternatively, bake in the oven at 400°F (200°C) for about 20-25 minutes.

Check for Doneness:

Ensure the tofu is cooked through and the vegetables have a slight char.

Serve:

Serve the Tofu and Vegetable Skewers hot as a standalone dish or over a bed of cooked quinoa or rice.

Enjoy!

Enjoy these flavorful and protein-packed skewers as a wholesome vegetarian meal.

Note: Feel free to customize the vegetables based on your preferences. You can also add a drizzle of lemon juice or a sprinkle of fresh herbs before serving.

Nutrition Information (Per Serving):

• Calories: 250

• Protein: 15g

• Fat: 12g

• Carbohydrates: 20g

• Fiber: 4g

• Sugar: 8g

EGG WHITE OMELETTE WITH SPINACH AND TOMATOES

Meal Description: The Egg White Omelette with Spinach and Tomatoes is a light and healthy breakfast option that provides a protein-packed start to your day. This omelette is filled with the freshness of spinach and tomatoes, creating a flavorful and nutrient-rich morning dish.

Ingredients:

- 1 cup egg whites (about six large egg whites)

- 1 cup fresh spinach, chopped

- 1/2 cup cherry tomatoes, halved

- 1/4 cup red onion, finely chopped

- One clove of garlic, minced

- One tablespoon of olive oil

- Salt and black pepper to taste

- Optional: Feta cheese or goat cheese for garnish

- Fresh herbs (such as parsley or chives) for garnish

Instructions:

Prepare Vegetables:

Chop the fresh spinach, halve the cherry tomatoes, and finely chop the red onion and garlic.

Sauté Vegetables:

In a non-stick skillet, heat olive oil over medium heat. Add red onion and garlic, sautéing until softened.

Add Spinach and Tomatoes:

Add chopped spinach and halved cherry tomatoes to the skillet. Cook for 2-3 minutes until the spinach wilts and the tomatoes soften slightly. Season with salt and black pepper.

Set Vegetables Aside:

Remove the sautéed vegetables from the skillet and set them aside in a bowl.

Whisk Egg Whites:

In a separate bowl, whisk the egg whites until frothy.

Cook Egg Whites:

Pour the whisked egg whites into the same skillet over medium heat. Allow them to sit for a moment.

Add Vegetables:

Add the sautéed spinach, tomatoes, and onions on one half of the omelette as the edges of the egg whites set.

Fold and Cook:

Gently fold the other half of the omelette over the vegetables, creating a half-moon shape. Cook for an additional 2-3 minutes until the omelette is fully set.

Optional Cheese:

If desired, crumble some feta cheese or goat cheese over the omelette during the last minute of cooking.

Garnish and Serve:

Garnish the Egg White Omelette with Spinach and Tomatoes with fresh herbs. Slide it onto a plate.

Enjoy!

Enjoy this light and nutritious omelette as a wholesome breakfast or brunch.

Nutrition Information (Per Serving):

• Calories: 150

• Protein: 25g

• Fat: 6g

• Carbohydrates: 5g

• Fiber: 2g

• Sugar: 2g

BAKED COD WITH GARLIC AND LEMON

Meal Description: Baked Cod with Garlic and Lemon is a simple and flavorful dish that highlights the natural taste of cod while enhancing it with the zesty brightness of lemon and the savoury aroma of garlic. This light and healthy recipe is easy to prepare, making it perfect for a quick and delicious seafood dinner.

Ingredients:

• Four cod fillets (about 6 oz each)

• Three tablespoons olive oil

• Four cloves garlic, minced

• Zest of 1 lemon

• Juice of 1 lemon

• One teaspoon of dried thyme

• One teaspoon paprika

• Salt and black pepper to taste

• Fresh parsley for garnish

• Lemon slices for serving

Instructions:

Preheat Oven:

Preheat the oven to 400°F (200°C).

Prepare Cod Fillets:

Pat the cod fillets dry with paper towels and place them in a baking dish.

Create Garlic and Lemon Marinade:

Whisk together olive oil, minced garlic, lemon zest, lemon juice, dried thyme, paprika, salt, and black pepper in a small bowl.

Marinate Cod:

Pour the marinade over the cod fillets, ensuring they are well coated. Let them marinate for at least 15 minutes to absorb the flavours.

Bake:

Bake the cod fillets in the preheated oven for 12-15 minutes or until the fish flakes easily with a fork. The cooking time may vary based on the thickness of the fillets.

Broil for Crispy Top (Optional):

For a slightly crispy top, you can broil the cod for an additional 1-2 minutes until the top is golden brown.

Check for Doneness:

Ensure the cod is cooked through and the internal temperature reaches 145°F (63°C).

Garnish:

Garnish the Baked Cod with Garlic and Lemon with

fresh parsley.

Serve:

Serve the cod fillets hot with lemon slices for an extra burst of citrus flavour.

Enjoy!

Enjoy this simple and delightful Baked Cod with Garlic and Lemon as a light, healthy seafood dinner.

Nutrition Information (Per Serving):

- Calories: 250
- Protein: 30g
- Fat: 12g
- Carbohydrates: 2g
- Fiber: 1g
- Sugar: 0g

SHRIMP AND QUINOA SALAD

Meal Description: Shrimp and Quinoa Salad is a refreshing and protein-packed dish that combines the succulence of shrimp with the nutty flavour of quinoa, all tossed with crisp vegetables and a zesty dressing. This salad is delicious and a satisfying and wholesome option for a light lunch or dinner.

Ingredients:

• 1 cup quinoa, rinsed and cooked according to package instructions

• 1 pound shrimp, peeled and deveined

• Two tablespoons of olive oil

• One teaspoon of smoked paprika

• One teaspoon of garlic powder

• Salt and black pepper to taste

Vegetable Mix:

• 1 cup cherry tomatoes, halved

• One cucumber, diced

• One bell pepper (any colour), diced

• 1/4 cup red onion, finely chopped

• 1/4 cup fresh parsley, chopped

Dressing:

• Three tablespoons olive oil

• Two tablespoons of red wine vinegar

• Juice of 1 lemon

• One teaspoon of Dijon mustard

• Salt and black pepper to taste

Instructions:

Cook Quinoa:

Rinse quinoa under cold water and cook it according to the package instructions. Once cooked, fluff the quinoa with a fork and let it cool.

Prepare Shrimp:

Toss shrimp with olive oil, smoked paprika, garlic powder, salt, and black pepper in a bowl. Heat a skillet over medium-high heat and cook the shrimp for 2-3 minutes per side or until they are opaque and cooked through.

Prepare Vegetables:

Combine the cooked quinoa with cherry tomatoes, cucumber, bell pepper, red onion, and fresh parsley in a large salad bowl.

Make Dressing:

Whisk together olive oil, red wine vinegar, lemon juice, Dijon mustard, salt, and black pepper in a small bowl.

Assemble Salad:

Add the cooked shrimp to the salad bowl. Drizzle the dressing over the salad and toss everything gently to combine.

Chill (Optional):

For enhanced flavours, you can chill the shrimp and quinoa salad in the refrigerator for 30 minutes before serving.

Serve:

Serve the Shrimp and Quinoa Salad in individual bowls or on a platter.

Enjoy!

Enjoy this light and nutritious salad as a satisfying meal or a delightful side dish.

Nutrition Information (Per Serving):

• Calories: 350

• Protein: 25g

• Fat: 18g

• Carbohydrates: 30g

• Fiber: 4g

• Sugar: 3g

GRILLED CHICKEN AND VEGGIE KEBABS

Meal Description: Grilled Chicken and Veggie Kebabs are a tasty and wholesome barbecue or outdoor meal option. Marinated chicken chunks are threaded onto skewers along with colourful vegetables, creating a delightful combination of flavours and textures. This recipe is perfect for a healthy and satisfying dinner straight from the grill.

Ingredients:

• 1.5 pounds boneless, skinless chicken breasts cut into chunks

• One zucchini, sliced into rounds

• One red bell pepper, cut into chunks

• One yellow bell pepper, cut into chunks

• One red onion, cut into chunks

• Cherry tomatoes

• Wooden skewers soaked in water for at least 30 minutes

Marinade:

• 1/4 cup olive oil

- Two tablespoons of balsamic vinegar

- Two cloves garlic, minced

- One teaspoon dried oregano

- One teaspoon of dried thyme

- One teaspoon of smoked paprika

- Salt and black pepper to taste

Instructions:

Prepare Marinade:

Whisk together olive oil, balsamic vinegar, minced garlic, dried oregano, dried thyme, smoked paprika, salt, and black pepper to create the marinade.

Marinate Chicken:

Place the chicken chunks in a shallow dish and coat them with half of the marinade. Allow the chicken to marinate for at least 30 minutes, refrigerate.

Preheat Grill:

Preheat the grill to medium-high heat.

Assemble Kebabs:

Thread the marinated chicken chunks, zucchini slices, red and yellow bell pepper chunks, red onion chunks, and cherry tomatoes onto the soaked wooden skewers, alternating the ingredients.

Brush with Marinade:

Brush the assembled kebabs with the remaining marinade for added flavour.

Grill:

Place the kebabs on the preheated grill and cook for 10-15 minutes, turning occasionally, until the chicken is cooked through and the vegetables are tender with a slight char.

Check for Doneness:

Ensure the chicken reaches an internal temperature of 165°F (74°C).

Serve:

Carefully remove the Grilled Chicken and Veggie Kebabs from the skewers and arrange them on a serving platter.

Enjoy!

Enjoy these delicious kebabs as a flavorful and nutritious meal for outdoor gatherings.

Note: Customize the vegetables based on your preference, and serve the kebabs with your favourite sauce or dip.

Nutrition Information (Per Serving):

• Calories: 300

• Protein: 30g

• Fat: 15g

• Carbohydrates: 15g

• Fiber: 4g

• Sugar: 8g

CHAPTER SIX

Healthy Fats Recipes

Avocado Toast With Tomatoes

Meal Description: Avocado Toast with Tomatoes is a simple yet satisfying dish that combines creamy avocado with juicy tomatoes on a bed of toasted bread. This open-faced sandwich is delicious and a nutrient-packed option for a quick and healthy breakfast or snack.

Ingredients:

• Two slices of whole-grain bread (or bread of your choice)

• One ripe avocado

• 1 cup cherry tomatoes, sliced

• One tablespoon of olive oil

• Salt and black pepper to taste

• Optional toppings: Red pepper flakes, crushed feta, or a sprinkle of chives

Instructions:

Toast-Bread:

Toast the slices of bread to your desired level of crispiness.

Prepare Avocado:

While the bread is toasting, cut the ripe avocado in half, remove the pit, and scoop the flesh into a bowl.

Mash Avocado:

Mash the avocado with a fork until smooth. Season

with salt and black pepper to taste.

Slice Tomatoes:

Slice the cherry tomatoes into thin rounds.

Assemble Avocado Toast:

Spread the mashed avocado evenly onto the toasted bread slices.

Add Tomatoes:

Arrange the sliced cherry tomatoes on top of the mashed avocado.

Drizzle Olive Oil:

Drizzle olive oil over the avocado and tomatoes.

Season:

Season the Avocado Toast with Tomatoes with a pinch of salt and black pepper.

Optional Toppings:

If desired, sprinkle red pepper flakes, crushed feta, or chives on top for added flavour.

Serve:

Serve the Avocado Toast with Tomatoes immediately.

Enjoy!

Enjoy this delicious, nutritious, open-faced sandwich as a quick, wholesome breakfast or snack.

Note: Feel free to customize the recipe by adding poached or fried eggs on top for extra protein.

Nutrition Information (Per Serving):

- Calories: 300
- Protein: 8g
- Fat: 20g
- Carbohydrates: 25g
- Fiber: 8g
- Sugar: 3g

SALMON AND AVOCADO SALAD

Meal Description: Salmon and Avocado Salad is a delightful and nutrient-rich dish that combines the heart-healthy benefits of salmon with the creamy texture of avocado. This salad is delicious and packed with omega-3 fatty acids, making it a perfect choice for a light and fulfilling lunch or dinner.

Ingredients:

• 1 pound salmon fillets, cooked and flaked

• Two ripe avocados, diced

• 2 cups mixed salad greens (arugula, spinach, or your choice)

• 1 cup cherry tomatoes, halved

• 1/4 cup red onion, thinly sliced

• One cucumber, sliced

• 1/4 cup feta cheese, crumbled

• Two tablespoons of olive oil

• Juice of 1 lemon

• One tablespoon of balsamic vinegar

• Salt and black pepper to taste

• Fresh dill for garnish

Instructions:

Prepare Salmon:

Cook the salmon fillets through your preferred method (grilling, baking, or pan-searing). Once cooked, flake the salmon into bite-sized pieces.

Assemble Salad:

Combine the mixed salad greens, diced avocado, halved cherry tomatoes, sliced red onion, cucumber slices, and flaked salmon in a large salad bowl.

Add Feta Cheese:

Sprinkle crumbled feta cheese over the salad ingredients.

Make Dressing:

Whisk together olive oil, lemon juice, balsamic vinegar, salt, and black pepper in a small bowl to create the dressing.

Toss Salad:

Drizzle the dressing over the salad and toss gently to coat all ingredients evenly.

Check Seasoning:

Taste and adjust the seasoning if necessary. Add more salt or pepper, according to your preference.

Garnish:

Garnish the Salmon and Avocado Salad with fresh dill for a burst of herbaceous flavour.

Serve:

Divide the salad into individual bowls or plates.

Enjoy!

Enjoy this wholesome and flavorful Salmon and Avocado Salad as a light and nutritious meal.

Note: Customize the salad by adding additional vegetables, nuts, or seeds for extra crunch and variety.

Nutrition Information (Per Serving):

• Calories: 400

• Protein: 25g

• Fat: 28g

• Carbohydrates: 15g

• Fiber: 8g

• Sugar: 3g

WALNUT AND MIXED GREENS SALAD

Meal Description: Walnut and Mixed Greens Salad is a delightful and nutritious dish that combines the earthy flavour of mixed greens with the crunch of walnuts and the sweetness of dried fruits. Tossed in a tangy vinaigrette, this salad is delicious and a perfect side or light meal.

Ingredients:

• 4 cups mixed salad greens (arugula, spinach, romaine, etc.)

• 1 cup walnuts, roughly chopped

• 1/2 cup dried cranberries or raisins

• 1/4 cup red onion, thinly sliced

• 1/2 cup crumbled feta cheese

• One apple, thinly sliced

• Two tablespoons extra-virgin olive oil

• One tablespoon of balsamic vinegar

• One teaspoon of Dijon mustard

• One teaspoon of honey or maple syrup

• Salt and black pepper to taste

Instructions:

Prepare Salad Greens:

Wash and dry the mixed salad greens thoroughly. Place them in a large salad bowl.

Add Walnuts:

Sprinkle the roughly chopped walnuts over the mixed greens.

Include Dried Fruits:

Add dried cranberries or raisins to the salad.

Slice Red Onion:

Thinly slice the red onion and add it to the salad.

Incorporate Feta Cheese:

Sprinkle crumbled feta cheese over the salad ingredients.

Add Sliced Apple:

Thinly slice the apple and incorporate it into the salad for a touch of sweetness.

Make Vinaigrette:

Whisk together extra-virgin olive oil, balsamic vinegar, Dijon mustard, honey or maple syrup, salt, and black pepper in a small bowl to create the vinaigrette.

Toss Salad:

Drizzle the vinaigrette over the salad and toss gently to coat all ingredients evenly.

Check Seasoning:

Taste and adjust the seasoning if necessary. Add more salt, pepper, or a touch of honey if desired.

Serve:

Serve the Walnut and Mixed Greens Salad on individual plates or as a side dish.

Enjoy!

Enjoy this vibrant and flavorful salad as a refreshing and nutrient-packed addition to your meal.

Note: Feel free to customize the salad by adding grilled chicken or chickpeas for added protein.

Nutrition Information (Per Serving):

• Calories: 350

• Protein: 8g

• Fat: 28g

• Carbohydrates: 20g

• Fiber: 5g

• Sugar: 12g

OLIVE OIL AND BALSAMIC ROASTED BRUSSELS SPROUTS

Meal Description: Olive Oil and Balsamic Roasted Brussels Sprouts are a delicious and flavorful side dish that transforms these cruciferous vegetables into crispy, caramelized bites. This simple recipe enhances the natural sweetness of Brussels sprouts with the richness of olive oil and the tanginess of balsamic vinegar, creating a perfect balance of flavours.

Ingredients:

- 1 pound Brussels sprouts, trimmed and halved
- Two tablespoons of olive oil
- Two tablespoons of balsamic vinegar
- One teaspoon of honey or maple syrup
- Two cloves garlic, minced
- Salt and black pepper to taste

- Optional: Grated Parmesan cheese for garnish
- Optional: Chopped fresh parsley for garnish

Instructions:

Preheat Oven:

Preheat the oven to 400°F (200°C).

Prepare Brussels Sprouts:

Trim the Brussels sprouts, remove any loose outer leaves, and cut them in half.

Make Marinade:

Whisk together olive oil, balsamic vinegar, honey or maple syrup, minced garlic, salt, and black pepper in a bowl to create the marinade.

Coat Brussels Sprouts:

Toss the halved Brussels sprouts in the marinade, ensuring they are well coated.

Roast in the Oven:

Spread the Brussels sprouts in a single layer on a baking sheet. Roast in the oven for 20-25 minutes or until golden brown and crispy on the edges.

Check for Doneness:

Pierce a Brussels sprout with a fork to ensure it's tender on the inside.

Optional Garnishes:

If desired, sprinkle grated Parmesan cheese and chopped fresh parsley over the roasted Brussels sprouts before serving.

Serve:

Transfer the Olive Oil and Balsamic Roasted Brussels Sprouts to a serving dish.

Enjoy!

Enjoy this flavorful and healthy side dish as a complement to your favourite main courses.

Note: Adjust the roasting time based on the size of the Brussels sprouts, and be sure to toss them halfway through for even cooking.

Nutrition Information (Per Serving):

• Calories: 120

• Protein: 4g

• Fat: 7g

• Carbohydrates: 14g

• Fiber: 4g

• Sugar: 4g

ALMOND-CRUSTED TILAPIA

Meal Description: Almond-crusted Tilapia is a delightful and nutritious dish that adds a crunchy twist to mild tilapia fillets. The combination of almond crust and flavorful seasonings creates a tasty coating that complements the tender tilapia. This recipe is easy to prepare and perfect for a light and satisfying dinner.

Ingredients:

• Four tilapia fillets

• 1 cup almonds, finely chopped or ground

• 1/2 cup breadcrumbs (whole wheat for a healthier option)

• One teaspoon of garlic powder

• One teaspoon of onion powder

• One teaspoon paprika

• 1/2 teaspoon dried thyme

• Salt and black pepper to taste

• Two eggs, beaten

• Olive oil for pan-frying

Instructions:

Preheat Oven:

Preheat the oven to 375°F (190°C).

Prepare Coating:

Combine finely chopped or ground almonds, breadcrumbs, garlic powder, onion powder, paprika, dried thyme, salt, and black pepper in a shallow dish. Mix well to create the almond crust.

Coat Tilapia Fillets:

Dip each tilapia fillet into the beaten eggs, ensuring it is fully coated.

Apply Almond Crust:

Press the egg-coated tilapia fillet into the almond crust mixture, covering both sides evenly. Gently pat the almond mixture onto the fillet to adhere.

Pan-Fry Tilapia:

Heat olive oil in a skillet over medium heat. Pan-fry the almond-crusted tilapia fillets on each side for 2-3 minutes until golden brown.

Transfer to Oven:

Transfer the partially cooked tilapia fillets to a baking sheet. Finish cooking them in the preheated oven for an additional 10-12 minutes or until the fish is opaque and flakes easily.

Check for Doneness:

Ensure the internal temperature of the Tilapia reaches 145°F (63°C).

Serve:

Serve the Almond-Crusted Tilapia hot, garnished

with fresh herbs if desired.

Enjoy!

Enjoy this flavorful and crunchy Almond-Crusted Tilapia as a delicious and wholesome main course.

Note: Adjust the cooking time based on the thickness of the tilapia fillets.

Nutrition Information (Per Serving):

- Calories: 300

- Protein: 25g

- Fat: 18g

- Carbohydrates: 10g

- Fiber: 4g

- Sugar: 1g

GUACAMOLE WITH VEGGIE STICKS

Meal Description: Guacamole with Veggie Sticks is a classic and nutritious snack that combines the creamy goodness of avocados with the freshness of assorted vegetables. This recipe yields a flavorful and satisfying dip, perfect for dipping crunchy veggie sticks. It's an excellent choice for a wholesome appetizer or a light, guilt-free snack.

Ingredients:

• Three ripe avocados

• One medium tomato, diced

• 1/2 red onion, finely chopped

• One jalapeño pepper, seeded and minced (optional for heat)

• 1/4 cup fresh cilantro, chopped

• Two cloves garlic, minced

• Juice of 1 lime

• Salt and black pepper to taste

• Assorted vegetable sticks (carrots, cucumber, bell peppers) for dipping

Instructions:

Prepare Avocados:

Cut the avocados in half, remove the pits, and scoop the flesh into a bowl.

Mash Avocados:

Mash the avocados with a fork or potato masher until you achieve your desired level of creaminess.

Add Ingredients:

Add diced tomatoes, finely chopped red onion, minced jalapeño (if using), chopped cilantro, minced garlic, and lime juice to the mashed avocados.

Season:

Season the guacamole with salt and black pepper to taste. Mix well to combine all the ingredients.

Adjust Consistency:

Adjust the consistency by adding more lime juice for acidity or more salt to enhance the flavour.

Chill (Optional):

For enhanced flavours, you can chill the guacamole in the refrigerator for about 30 minutes before serving.

Prepare Veggie Sticks:

Wash and cut assorted vegetables into sticks. Common choices include carrots, cucumber, and bell peppers.

Serve:

Transfer the guacamole to a serving bowl, surround it with the veggie sticks, and arrange them on a platter.

Enjoy!

Enjoy this delightful Guacamole with Veggie Sticks as a healthy and satisfying snack.

Note: Customize the level of spiciness by adjusting the amount of jalapeño used.

Nutrition Information (Per Serving):

• Calories: 200

• Protein: 4g

• Fat: 15g

• Carbohydrates: 18g

• Fiber: 10g

• Sugar: 3g

PESTO ZUCCHINI NOODLES

Meal Description: Pesto Zucchini Noodles are a light and flavorful alternative to traditional pasta, featuring spiralized zucchini tossed in a vibrant and herbaceous pesto sauce. This dish is not only delicious but also low in carbs and high in nutrients, making it a perfect choice for a quick and healthy meal.

Ingredients:

For the Pesto:

• 2 cups fresh basil leaves, packed

• 1/2 cup grated Parmesan cheese

• 1/2 cup pine nuts or walnuts

• Two cloves garlic, minced

• 1/2 cup extra-virgin olive oil

• Salt and black pepper to taste

For the Zucchini Noodles:

• Four medium-sized zucchini, spiralized

• One tablespoon of olive oil

• Salt and black pepper to taste

• Optional: Cherry tomatoes and extra Parmesan for

garnish

Instructions:

Prepare Pesto:

Combine fresh basil, grated Parmesan cheese, pine nuts or walnuts, and minced garlic in a food processor.

Pulse the ingredients until coarsely chopped.

With the food processor running, gradually add the olive oil in a steady stream until the pesto reaches your desired consistency.

Season with salt and black pepper to taste. Set aside.

Prepare Zucchini Noodles:

Spiralize the zucchini using a spiralizer to create noodles.

Heat olive oil in a large skillet over medium heat.

Add the zucchini noodles to the skillet and sauté for 2-3 minutes until they are just tender but still have a slight crunch.

Season the zucchini noodles with salt and black pepper to taste.

Combine Pesto and Zucchini Noodles:

Add the prepared pesto to the skillet with zucchini noodles.

Toss the noodles until they are evenly coated with the pesto sauce.

Cook for an additional 1-2 minutes to warm the pesto.

Serve:

Transfer the Pesto Zucchini Noodles to a serving

platter or individual plates.

Garnish with cherry tomatoes and additional grated Parmesan if desired.

Enjoy! Indulge in this light and delicious Pesto Zucchini Noodles dish as a nutritious and satisfying alternative to traditional pasta.

Note: Feel free to add grilled chicken, shrimp, or your favourite protein for an extra boost of protein.

Nutrition Information (Per Serving):

• Calories: 250

• Protein: 7g

• Fat: 22g

• Carbohydrates: 10g

• Fiber: 4g

• Sugar: 4g

CHIA SEED PUDDING WITH BERRIES

Meal Description: Chia Seed Pudding with Berries is a delightful and nutritious dessert or breakfast option that combines chia seeds' richness with fresh berries' sweetness. This simple recipe allows you to create a creamy and satisfying pudding that's delicious and packed with omega-3 fatty acids and antioxidants.

Ingredients:

For the Chia Seed Pudding:

• 1/4 cup chia seeds

• 1 cup almond milk (or any milk of your choice)

• One tablespoon of maple syrup or honey

• 1/2 teaspoon vanilla extract

For Topping:

• Mixed berries (strawberries, blueberries, raspberries)

• Optional toppings: Sliced almonds, shredded coconut, or a drizzle of additional maple syrup

Instructions:

Prepare Chia Seed Pudding:

1. Combine chia seeds, almond milk, maple syrup (or honey), and vanilla extract in a bowl.

2. Whisk the ingredients together until well combined.

3. Let the mixture sit for 5 minutes, then whisk again to prevent clumping.

4. Cover the bowl and refrigerate for at least 2 hours or overnight to allow the chia seeds to absorb the liquid and create a pudding-like consistency.

Assemble Chia Seed Pudding with Berries:

1. Once the chia pudding has set, give it a good stir to ensure a smooth texture.

2. Spoon the chia seed pudding into serving bowls or jars.

Add Berries:

1. Top the chia seed pudding with a generous amount of mixed berries.

2. Feel free to mix and match different berries for a colourful and flavorful topping.

Optional Toppings:

1. Sprinkle sliced almonds or shredded coconut on top for added crunch.

2. Drizzle a bit of additional maple syrup for extra sweetness, if desired.

Serve: Serve the Chia Seed Pudding with Berries immediately as a refreshing and wholesome dessert or breakfast option.

Enjoy! Indulge in the delightful combination of creamy chia seed pudding and fresh, juicy berries for a nutritious and satisfying treat.

Nutrition Information (Per Serving):

- Calories: 200

- Protein: 5g

- Fat: 10g

- Carbohydrates: 25g

- Fiber: 10g

- Sugar: 10g

FLAXSEED AND BANANA SMOOTHIE

Meal Description: The Flaxseed and Banana Smoothie is a nutritious and energy-boosting beverage that combines the natural sweetness of bananas with the health benefits of flaxseeds. Packed with omega-3 fatty acids, fibre, and essential nutrients, this smoothie is delicious and a great way to kickstart your day or replenish your energy post-workout.

Ingredients:

• Two ripe bananas, peeled and sliced

• One tablespoon of ground flaxseeds

• 1 cup Greek yoghurt (or dairy-free alternative)

• 1/2 cup almond milk (or any milk of your choice)

• One tablespoon honey (optional for added sweetness)

• Ice cubes (optional)

• Optional toppings: Sliced bananas, a sprinkle of flaxseeds, or a drizzle of honey

Instructions:

Prepare Ingredients:

Peel and slice the ripe bananas.

Blend Smoothie:

In a blender, combine the sliced bananas, ground flaxseeds, Greek yoghurt, almond milk, and honey (if using).

Blend the ingredients until smooth and creamy.

Adjust Consistency:

Add more almond milk or water to reach your desired consistency if the smoothie is too thick.

Add Ice Cubes (Optional):

For a colder and more refreshing smoothie, add a handful of ice cubes to the blender and blend until the ice is fully incorporated.

Serve:

Pour the Flaxseed and Banana Smoothie into glasses.

Optional Toppings:

Garnish the smoothie with sliced bananas, a sprinkle of flaxseeds, or a drizzle of honey, if desired.

Enjoy! Savour the creamy and nutrient-packed goodness of the Flaxseed and Banana Smoothie as a delicious and wholesome drink.

Nutrition Information (Per Serving):

• Calories: 300

• Protein: 15g

• Fat: 8g

• Carbohydrates: 45g

• Fiber: 8g

• Sugar: 25g

HUMMUS WITH OLIVE TAPENADE

Meal Description: Hummus with Olive Tapenade is a flavorful and Mediterranean-inspired dip that combines the creamy texture of Hummus with the briny goodness of olive tapenade. This dish is perfect for entertaining, serving as an appetizer, or enjoying as a delicious and wholesome snack.

Ingredients:

For the Hummus:

• One can (15 ounces) chickpeas, drained and rinsed

• 1/4 cup tahini

• Two tablespoons of olive oil

• Two cloves garlic, minced

• Juice of 1 lemon

• 1/2 teaspoon ground cumin

• Salt and black pepper to taste

• Water (as needed for desired consistency)

For the Olive Tapenade:

• 1 cup mixed olives (Kalamata, green, black), pitted and chopped

- Two tablespoons capers, drained and chopped
- One tablespoon of fresh parsley chopped
- One tablespoon of olive oil
- Juice of 1/2 lemon
- One clove of garlic, minced
- Black pepper to taste

For Serving:

- Drizzle of olive oil
- Fresh parsley for garnish
- Pita bread, sliced vegetables, or crackers for dipping

Instructions:

Prepare Hummus:

1. Combine chickpeas, tahini, olive oil, minced garlic, lemon juice, ground cumin, salt, and black pepper in a food processor.

2. Blend the ingredients until smooth, adding water as needed to achieve your desired hummus consistency.

Prepare Olive Tapenade:

1. Combine chopped olives, capers, fresh parsley, olive oil, lemon juice, minced garlic, and black pepper in a bowl.

2. Mix the ingredients well to create the olive tapenade.

Assemble Hummus with Olive Tapenade:

1. Spoon the Hummus onto a serving plate, creating a well in the centre.

2. Fill the well with the olive tapenade, spreading it evenly over the Hummus.

Serve:

1. Drizzle a bit of olive oil over the top.

2. Garnish with fresh parsley.

3. Serve the Hummus with Olive Tapenade with sliced pita bread, vegetables, or crackers for dipping.

Enjoy! Indulge in Hummus's rich and savoury combination with Olive tapenade as a delightful appetizer or snack with a Mediterranean flair.

Note: Customize the olive tapenade by adding ingredients like sun-dried tomatoes or roasted red peppers for additional flavour.

Nutrition Information (Per Serving):

• Calories: 250

• Protein: 8g

• Fat: 18g

• Carbohydrates: 20g

• Fiber: 6g

• Sugar: 2g

CHAPTER SEVEN

Hydration Recipes

Cucumber And Lemon Detox Water

Beverage Description: Cucumber and Lemon Detox Water is a refreshing and hydrating drink that combines the natural flavours of cucumber and lemon, providing a burst of citrusy and cooling goodness. This detox water is not only delicious but also an excellent way to stay hydrated while enjoying the potential benefits of detoxification.

Ingredients:

• One cucumber, thinly sliced

• One lemon, thinly sliced

• 2-3 sprigs of fresh mint (optional)

• 8 cups water (filtered or still mineral water)

• Ice cubes (optional)

Instructions:

Prepare Ingredients:

1. Wash the cucumber and lemon thoroughly.

2. Cut the cucumber and lemon into thin slices.

Assemble Detox Water:

1. Combine the cucumber slices, lemon slices, and fresh mint sprigs in a large pitcher.

2. Fill the pitcher with 8 cups of water.

3. If desired, add ice cubes to make the detox water extra refreshing.

Infuse:

1. Allow the ingredients to infuse in the refrigerator for at least 2 hours or overnight for enhanced flavour.

2. The longer the water sits, the more invested and flavorful it will become.

Serve:

1. Pour the Cucumber and Lemon Detox Water into glasses.

2. Garnish with additional cucumber or lemon slices and mint, if desired.

Enjoy! Sip on this revitalizing Cucumber and Lemon Detox Water throughout the day to stay hydrated and enjoy the refreshing taste of natural ingredients.

Note: Detox water is a great way to increase water intake and may have potential health benefits, including supporting hydration and providing a dose of antioxidants.

Nutrition Information (Per Serving):

• Calories: 0 (water-based)

• The ingredients add no significant macronutrients or calories.

PINEAPPLE COCONUT WATER

Beverage Description: Pineapple Coconut Water is a tropical and hydrating beverage that combines the sweet and tangy flavour of pineapple with the refreshing taste of coconut water. This drink is delicious and a natural source of hydration with added nutrients, making it a perfect choice for a revitalizing and thirst-quenching experience.

Ingredients:

• 2 cups fresh pineapple chunks

• 2 cups coconut water (new or packaged)

• Ice cubes (optional)

• Pineapple slices and mint leaves for garnish (optional)

Instructions:

Prepare Ingredients:

1. Peel and chop fresh pineapple into chunks.

Blend Pineapple and Coconut Water:

1. In a blender, combine fresh pineapple chunks and coconut water.

2. Blend until the mixture is smooth and well combined.

Strain (Optional):

1. If desired, strain the pineapple-coconut mixture to remove the pulp. This step is optional, as some may prefer the added fibre.

Chill:

1. Refrigerate the Pineapple Coconut Water for at least 1 hour to enhance the flavours and chill the drink.

Serve:

1. Pour the chilled Pineapple Coconut Water into glasses.

2. Add ice cubes if you prefer a colder beverage.

Garnish (Optional):

1. Garnish with pineapple slices and mint leaves for a decorative touch.

Enjoy! Savour the tropical goodness of Pineapple Coconut Water as a delightful and hydrating drink for any occasion.

Note: Coconut water is naturally rich in electrolytes, making it an excellent choice for rehydration. Pineapple adds natural sweetness and a dose of vitamin C.

Nutrition Information (Per Serving):

• Calories: 80

• Protein: 1g

• Fat: 0g

• Carbohydrates: 20g

• Fiber: 2g

• Sugar: 15g

HOMEMADE ELECTROLYTE DRINK

Beverage Description: A Homemade Electrolyte Drink is a natural and cost-effective way to replenish essential electrolytes, making it an ideal choice for rehydration after exercise, illness, or excessive heat. This DIY electrolyte drink provides a balance of sodium, potassium, and other minerals to support proper hydration and electrolyte balance.

Ingredients:

• 2 cups water (filtered or boiled and cooled)

• 1 cup coconut water

• Two tablespoons of honey or maple syrup

• 1/4 teaspoon salt (preferably sea salt)

• 1/4 teaspoon baking soda

• 1/2 teaspoon calcium magnesium powder (optional)

• Juice of 1 lemon or lime (about two tablespoons)

• Ice cubes (optional)

Instructions:

Prepare Ingredients:

1. Measure out the water, coconut water, honey or maple syrup, salt, baking soda, calcium magnesium powder (if using), and lemon or lime juice.

Mix Electrolyte Drink:

1. In a pitcher, combine the water and coconut water.

2. Add honey or maple syrup, salt, baking soda, and calcium magnesium powder (if using).

3. Squeeze the juice of one lemon or lime into the mixture.

4. Stir well to ensure all ingredients are thoroughly combined.

Chill (Optional):

1. Refrigerate the Homemade Electrolyte Drink for at least 1 hour to chill the mixture.

Serve:

1. Pour the Homemade Electrolyte Drink into glasses.

2. Add ice cubes if you prefer a colder beverage.

Enjoy! Rehydrate and replenish with this Homemade Electrolyte Drink, a natural and effective solution for maintaining electrolyte balance.

Note: This DIY electrolyte drink provides a balance of sodium, potassium, calcium, and magnesium, which are essential electrolytes for the body.

Nutrition Information (Per Serving):

• Calories: 80

• Protein: 0g

• Fat: 0g

• Carbohydrates: 20g

- Fibre: 0g
- Sugar: 18g

MANGO MINT LEMONADE

Beverage Description: Mango Mint Lemonade is a refreshing and tropical twist on classic lemonade, combining mango's sweet and luscious flavour with the zesty kick of fresh lemon juice and the invigorating essence of mint. This delightful drink is perfect for quenching your thirst on a hot day or serving as a vibrant party beverage.

Ingredients:

• 2 cups ripe mango, peeled and diced

• 1 cup fresh lemon juice (about 4-6 lemons)

• 1/2 cup mint leaves, loosely packed

• 1/2 cup honey or agave syrup (adjust to taste)

• 4 cups cold water

• Ice cubes

• Lemon slices and mint sprigs for garnish (optional)

Instructions:

Prepare Ingredients:

1. Peel and dice ripe mango.

2. Juice fresh lemons to obtain 1 cup of lemon juice.

3. Measure out mint leaves, honey, and cold water.

Blend Mango Mint Lemonade:

1. Combine diced mango, fresh lemon juice, mint leaves, and honey in a blender.

2. Blend until the mixture is smooth and well combined.

Strain (Optional):

1. If desired, strain the blended mixture to remove pulp and mint leaves. This step is optional, depending on your preference.

Mix and Chill:

1. In a large pitcher, combine the strained mixture with cold water.

2. Stir well to mix the ingredients thoroughly.

3. Refrigerate the Mango Mint Lemonade for at least 1-2 hours to enhance the flavours and chill the drink.

Serve:

1. Pour the chilled Mango Mint Lemonade into glasses.

2. Add ice cubes for extra refreshment.

Garnish (Optional):

1. Garnish each glass with a slice of lemon and a sprig of mint for a decorative touch.

Enjoy! Sip and savour the tropical delight of Mango Mint Lemonade, a vibrant and thirst-quenching beverage for any occasion.

Note: Adjust the sweetness by adding more or less honey or agave syrup to suit your taste preferences.

Nutrition Information (Per Serving):

- Calories: 120
- Protein: 1g
- Fat: 0g
- Carbohydrates: 30g
- Fiber: 2g
- Sugar: 26g

BLUEBERRY LAVENDER INFUSED WATER

Beverage Description: Blueberry Lavender Infused Water is a refreshing and aromatic drink that combines the sweet and antioxidant-rich flavour of blueberries with the subtle floral notes of lavender. This infused water provides a burst of natural flavours and a visually appealing and hydrating beverage without added sugars or artificial ingredients.

Ingredients:

• 1 cup fresh blueberries

• 2-3 sprigs of fresh lavender (or one teaspoon of dried lavender buds)

• 8 cups water (filtered or still mineral water)

• Ice cubes

• Optional: Lemon slices for extra freshness

Instructions:

Prepare Ingredients:

1. Wash the fresh blueberries and remove any stems.

2. Rinse the fresh lavender sprigs or measure out dried

lavender buds.

Infuse Blueberry Lavender Water:

1. In a large pitcher, combine fresh blueberries and lavender.

2. Fill the pitcher with 8 cups of water.

3. If desired, add ice cubes for a colder beverage.

Muddle (Optional):

1. Use a muddler or the back of a spoon to crush the blueberries and release their juices gently.

2. Be careful not to destroy the lavender too much to avoid a strong, bitter taste.

Chill:

1. Allow the Blueberry Lavender Infused Water to chill in the refrigerator for at least 2 hours, or preferably overnight, to intensify the flavours.

Serve:

1. Pour the infused water into glasses.

2. If desired, add lemon slices for an extra burst of freshness.

Enjoy! Sip and enjoy the delightful combination of Blueberry Lavender Infused Water, a visually appealing and hydrating drink with a hint of sweetness and floral aroma.

Note: Experiment with the lavender quantity to find the right balance of flavour, as lavender can have a strong taste.

Nutrition Information (Per Serving):

• Calories: 0 (water-based)

• The ingredients add no significant macronutrients or calories.

CONCLUSION

In conclusion, colon cancer stands as a formidable health challenge with far-reaching implications, affecting individuals across the globe. While numerous factors contribute to the development of this malignancy, the role of diet emerges as an adaptable and influential element in both prevention and management. The intricate relationship between what we consume and our risk of developing colon cancer underscores the importance of adopting a thoughtful and informed approach to dietary choices.

Evidence suggests that incorporating high-fiber foods, antioxidant-rich fruits and vegetables, and essential nutrients such as calcium and vitamin D can contribute to a lower risk of colon cancer. Conversely, the moderation of red and processed meat intake, selection of healthy fats, and responsible alcohol consumption are advocated as prudent measures in promoting colorectal health. The maintenance of a healthy weight, achieved through a balanced diet and regular physical activity, further underscores the interconnectedness of lifestyle choices and cancer risk.

However, it is crucial to recognize that dietary modifications are just one facet of a comprehensive colon cancer prevention and management strategy. Regular screenings, early detection, and personalized healthcare guidance are equally indispensable components of a holistic approach. The complexity of individual health profiles, genetic predispositions, and evolving medical research necessitate collaborative efforts between individuals, healthcare professionals, and researchers to refine our understanding and enhance preventive measures.

As we navigate the multifaceted landscape of colon cancer, it is evident that fostering awareness, making informed dietary decisions, and embracing a holistic approach to health is instrumental in our collective efforts to reduce the burden of this disease. By integrating the principles of a healthful diet into our lifestyles, we contribute to our individual well-being and participate in a broader movement towards a future where the impact of colon cancer is minimized and lives are prolonged and enriched.